TRANQUILLISATION: THE NON ADDICTIVE WAY

by

PHYLLIS SPEIGHT

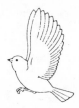

THE C. W. DANIEL COMPANY LIMITED
1 CHURCH PATH, SAFFRON WALDEN
ESSEX, ENGLAND

First published in Great Britain by
The C. W. Daniel Company Limited
1 Church Path, Saffron Walden
Essex CB10 1JP, England

ISBN 0 85207 228 7

Set by MS Typesetting, Castle Camps, Cambridge
and printed by Hillman Printers (Frome) Ltd,
Frome, Somerset, England

CONTENTS

INTRODUCTION

When I finished my previous book I decided that was it — no more — and I felt quite a sense of relief. After all, the ear, nose and throat are not parts of the body to get very excited about although they do give a lot of trouble.

My desk looked tidier than it had done for months and the odd bits of paper had been cleared away, pens and pencils put into place.

And then two things happened!

I met a dear person who asked me to help her stop taking Diazepam, one of the tranquillising drugs. Her husband had died 6 years ago and like many other people in the same circumstances, she said "I went to pieces". She saw her local doctor who was quite sympathetic in the short time he could spare to talk to her, and said she needed Diazepam. "Oh no, I don't want to take drugs" was her immediate response, but the doctor quickly tried to brush away her fears by saying, as he was writing out the prescription, "you have nothing to worry about, you don't have to see me more than once a year; when you need more tablets you can get a prescription from the surgery!"

The dose was 6 tablets daily. She had, however, reduced it to 4 but still had to take an extra one if she was anxious or worried about anything. This was after 6 years.

A day or two later a friend (and colleague) telephoned and in the course of conversation said "You'll never believe something that a patient told me this morning". She went on to relate how a new patient had made up her mind to have homoeopathic treatment because she was in a great state of anxiety and when she went to the doctor for help he prescribed Diazepam. "But I don't want to take drugs" said this patient. "I've heard dreadful things about them and about the side effects that they can produce." "Now" replied the doctor, "just think for a moment. If you suffered from diabetes you would have to take insulin, so I am giving you a tranquilliser." With that he handed her the prescription and that was the end of the conversation.

I cannot imagine the feelings of this poor woman but she was very grateful to sit quietly and give all her details to a caring homoeopath. I am sure she is now on the road to cure.

I couldn't forget these two happenings and my mind started to work in the direction of helping people to find another way of dealing with anxieties, grief, stress and the many conditions for which tranquillising drugs are prescribed automatically.

The *Observer* newspaper of the 17th December 1989 printed an article entitled "Drug firms face trial over pill addiction" by Annabel Ferriman and Tim Miles. It stated that writs are about to be served on the drug company giants Roche and Wyeth on behalf of some 2000 tranquilliser addicts. It also states that dozens of doctors who prescribed the drugs are also expected to face legal action.

The article goes on to say lawyers have been preparing the case for almost two years. They are expected to allege that the above mentioned companies failed to warn patients of the addictive nature of their products, in particular Valium and Ativan.

One complication is that people have switched from one brand of tranquilliser to another and after Valium and other branded drugs lost their patent protection people sometimes changed to the cheaper generic versions which are Diazepam and Chlordiazepoxide. The tendency to change was increased after the Department of Health banned the prescribing of Valium and Librium by name when it introduced a limited list of prescribable drugs in 1985, according to the article. The Department issued two warnings about the addictive nature of tranquillisers in 1980 and 1988 urging that they should be prescribed for shorter periods and fewer conditions!

There is little doubt that addiction to the tranquillising drugs has caused concern among some sufferers and it is hoped that this book will bring new hope and enable many to obtain relief by means of remedies that deal with the cause of the trouble and thus eliminate the need for drug therapy.

Another article in the *Daily Telegraph* (of 3rd January 1990) is headed "Tranquilliser Aid Agency to Close." It states that the leading agency Tranx UK., based at Wealdstone, North London, offering aid to people hooked on tranquillisers is to close later this month although it has a record number of inquiries from addicts who are desperate for help.

It has an established nationwide reputation, says the article, and has helped more than 86,000 people during the past 7 years but has now run out of money and cannot find another sponsor.

The article goes on to say "The Department of Health which provided the initial finance, says its money was a one-off grant and N.W. Thames

Health Authority which took over the funding along with other groups, says it can no longer finance a national organisation."

The correspondent continues "Miss Joan Jerome, who founded Tranx after being hooked on Valium and Mogadon said the prospect of closure was a 'terrific blow'. We receive 2,000 inquiries a month and have proved there is a vital need for the work we do. If we close now, we are cutting these people loose with no specialist help to turn to. Many of our clients could be driven to suicide."

This article helps to highlight the enormous size of the tranquilliser problem and it goes on to say that a Labour M.P. has contacted the Health Secretary to try and avert the agencies closure.

It seems ludicrous that doctors are allowed to prescribe drugs in this group, when so many patients appear to suffer far more from their side-effects than from the symptoms which took them to the G.P. for treatment in the first place.

Chapter 1

STRESS

*Find real health of mind and you will have gone
a long way towards finding health of body also.*
Norman Vincent Peale

Stress is probably the most common "disease"
there is. It is with us all the time. It crops up in
nearly everything we do; we see it in situations
on television; we read about it in the
newspapers. It is not surprising that a dis-
tinguished Canadian physician has advanced
the theory that "stress is an active agent in most
diseases".

The interesting thing about stress is the way
we react to it. That is the important part.

Out of stress arises anger, tension, anxiety,
fear, apprehension, insomnia, and other emotions, the list is a long one. We get tense when
doing things, the area round the back of the
neck and across the shoulders often taking the
brunt. We become impatient with people and
with ourselves; we become hurried, feeling that
everything must be done in a rush, and so on.
The end product is a very jaded system with
many varied symptoms.

I was horrified to see an example of this not
long ago when driving through our little town.
We stopped at traffic lights and I could see a

woman in the car behind us was in a state of agitation. Her hands were fidgeting, she was looking first in one direction, then in another, she was talking to herself which, of course, I couldn't hear. The lights changed and we drove off. At the top of the town the lights were red again and this time we pulled up alongside each other. We were at the cross-roads. She was going straight ahead and we were waiting to turn right. This woman was still talking to herself (swearing perhaps), tapping on the steering wheel, sighing and looked extremely het up. When the lights changed she shot across the road at high speed and was out of sight before we had turned the corner. I hope she never has an accident because other people might get hurt but I doubt very much whether she will escape a breakdown or physical illness if she repeats that performance of showing so much nervous tension (stress) too often.

The stupid part of that kind of behaviour which is not uncommon these days, is that it can only be harmful and cause more un-ease and stress.

Did you know that eating too much sugar can cause stress? I remember seeing a patient many years ago who was in a terrible state of anxiety. She always felt tired, had no energy yet she felt she had to rush to get things done which, of course, made matters worse.

When taking the case history I questioned her about her diet and after some pressure she admitted to taking lots of sugar every day − in fact her weekly intake was two pounds! She didn't need homoeopathic medicine but an adjustment in her diet and by cutting to the minimum sugar and sweet things she improved. After a month she was a different person and enjoying life with lots of energy.

Smoking is not good for us. It lowers the body's resistance and after a while many smokers develop a nasty cough. Substituting a cup of tea and a cigarette for a good meal not only becomes a bad habit but vital vitamins and minerals are leeched from the system and symptoms of stress get worse. So what happens when we take any drug that sedates or tranquillises the many aspects of stress?

The administration of these drugs makes us less able to cope with stresses that surround us by dulling our senses and filling our heads with cotton wool.

Remember that one of the reasons for writing this book was meeting the woman who had been taking Diazepam for the last 6 years following the death of her husband.

When I met her she had reduced the dose from 6 tablets to 4 but often had to take an extra dose, and I realized why. She was full of nervous movements, her hands always fidgeting; she smoked a lot, talked a great deal, was upset easily, fearing that she had said "the wrong thing" or should have done something different. Tears came easily but she was quickly comforted.

Here we have a patient full of anxiety, tension and fear (all parts of stress) and yet she had been taking the same drug for 6 years. Surely these were some of the symptoms that prompted the doctor to prescribe this drug in the first place?

From this we have to draw the conclusion that tranquillisers do nothing to cure the patient. Symptoms are suppressed and if events seem to get too much to cope with another dose is taken and life becomes just that bit more bearable again.

But that isn't quite the end of the story. These drugs develop side effects when taken for any length of time and they deprive the system of natural minerals and vitamins. But what is much more important, they weaken the immune system which means that the patient is more prone to virus infections, colds, winter ills and the recovery process takes far longer than it should. I have found on many occasions, when these aspects have been discussed, that very few people connect them, they seem to think they are all separate "happenings" in water-tight compartments.

Many people continue to take drugs for the rest of their lives, fearful of trying to reduce and finally give them up, because of what may happen, yet never gaining any real or lasting benefit from them.

The Daily Telegraph published an article (on 14th August 1989) stating that "High Street Chemists are to quiz customers who ask for tranquilliser prescriptions to be dispensed."

It goes on to say that pharmacists will be told to alert patients to the dangers of addiction because there is official concern at failure to reduce the 1,200,000 people addicted to benzodiazepines.

It is sad to think that problems for which patients are taking these drugs are not being tackled; if anything, by suppression they are being more deeply rooted in the economy of each person.

But there is light at the end of the tunnel. My second reason for writing this book was the woman who refused tranquillisers and sought homoeopathy.

We must now look into homoeopathy and what it has to offer.

Chapter 2

WHAT IS HOMOEOPATHY?

Homoeopathy is a complete system of medicine, used and taught in many countries, including our own.

There has been a homoeopathic physician attending our Royal Family for several generations.

The law of similars (recognised by Samuel Hahnemann who was born in 1755) is the corner-stone of homoeopathic prescribing – "let like be cured by like" – Similia Similibus Curentur.

This means that any substance that produces symptoms when taken by a healthy person will help to restore health to a sick patient exhibiting similar symptoms. (see "Proving Homoeopathic Remedies").

The next factor is the minute dose, the potentised remedies, as our medicines are called, and I have described this further on.

The patient is considered as a whole when prescribed for homoeopathically. By that I mean that of course the physical symptoms are taken into consideration, and in detail, but we believe that signs and symptoms are the outward manifestation that something is wrong at a much deeper level; that the life-force (which includes the immune system) has been disturbed and is not functioning as efficiently as it should.

This is why we match the remedy to the patient rather than to the part that is giving trouble and to do this we have to find out as much as we can about the person; how he reacts to weather, to foods, etc., but most important are the mind symptoms.

This is a vast subject and there are many books which give more details, but this brief explanation will, I hope, encourage more reading and also explain why I have mentioned so many times that the remedy must match the symptoms of the patient.

We can read a description of every disease that has a name but individuals react differently to Influenza, for instance. We have no "specific" medicine to cure Influenza but a choice of many remedies to cure patients who have developed symptoms that we call Influenza.

The booklist on page 96 will be of interest to those who wish to go more deeply into homoeopathy.

THE PROVING OF REMEDIES

In order to use a substance homoeopathically it must be tested and its range of action discovered and documented.

This is known as "proving".

Healthy volunteers take a substance under investigation on a regular basis until effects are produced. These effects are allowed to develop and are meticulously recorded; not only the physical changes but also mental and emotional changes.

Thus we have a complete "picture" of what the substance will do; and it will **cure** similar symptoms exhibited by a sick patient.

Hahnemann, his family and friends proved about 60 remedies. Today we have about 2,000 in our armoury and most of these have been fully proved.

I am happy to add that animals are never used for the testing of homoeopathic remedies. They cannot tell us how they feel, and they are different from human beings in so many ways.

Thus homoeopaths have a clear picture of the action of their remedies on humans and in addition, have the satisfaction of knowing that no suffering has been caused to animals.

THE PREPARATION OF
HOMOEOPATHIC REMEDIES

This is the most difficult part for people "outside" homoeopathy to understand.

Many have said that the cure or improvement is psychological because there is no medicinal substance in our remedies.

Homoeopathic remedies are potentised and I will endeavour to explain what we call "Potentisation".

The raw material of every substance used, whether animal, vegetable or mineral is made into a tincture, which we call the "mother tincture." If the substance is insoluble it is triturated with lactose (sugar of milk) according to disciplines laid down, and then dissolved in alcohol in order to obtain the mother tincture.

One drop of the mother tincture is then added to 99 drops of distilled water and shaken vigorously (this is called succussion). This produces the first centesimal potency shown as 1 or 1c. One drop of this is added to a further 99 drops of distilled water and succussed, this gives the second centesimal potency (2c). Succeeding potencies are prepared in the same manner. All homoeopathic remedies are available in a wide range of potencies; the 6c, 12c, 30c and 200c are in general use but much higher potencies are used by experienced homoeopaths.

There is another scale of preparation – the decimal potencies which are made in the same manner but one drop of the mother tincture is succussed with only 9 drops of distilled water; these potencies are denoted by the suffix "x": – 6x, 12x, 30x and so on or by the prefix "D"; D6, D12, D30 etc. They are more widely used on the continent than in the U.K.

Potencies of 12c and over do not contain a single molecule of the original substance yet the higher the potency the greater its strength as each succussion releases more healing power. This fact is being demonstrated every day as experienced practitioners prescribe the high potencies. I hope that at some further date instruments will be constructed which will give indisputable proof of the presence of this amazing power which seems impossible to materialists who do not accept any fact without proof.

Chapter 3

MIND STATES

I have discussed, in the following pages, some of the more common states of mind that are very prevalent to-day.

Patents complaining of anxiety, depression, fear and so on, arrive in the consulting room of every therapist far too frequently.

I had my share and always felt thankful that homoeopathy would help; very often there were deep rooted problems to sort out.

It is not difficult to understand how so many of these patients get hooked on tranquillisers.

When a person feels that she cannot cope with her problems any longer she decides to consult her G.P. After waiting in a crowded room for some time she is called into the surgery where she finds it difficult to describe her symptoms. Before she has finished the doctor is already writing a prescription – he has seen all this before and knows what is required. The long trail on drugs has begun; repeat prescriptions are readily available.

At this point I must say that, generally, I'm sure doctors are sincere in wanting to do all they can for their patients. And it is very encouraging to meet more and more who are, at least, sufficiently open-minded to acknowledge that there are other ways of treating the sick.

What I feel very strongly about, and I know that many people agree, is the system in which the allopathic physician has to work. With a couple of thousand patients on his list and illness all around, 7 or 8 minutes is, very often all that he can give to each patient.

But worse than that the choice of treatment is limited to drugs and drugs create trouble in the long term.

We should remember that the drug houses — who are out to make as much money as possible — are working flat out to produce "better" and "more efficient" drugs to combat disease. This means that each one becomes more powerful than the last and so the side-effects become more numerous and more difficult to cope with. More power = more danger.

The doctors are warned against all these pitfalls — the warnings are published in a booklet, but the mind boggles at the idea of any group practitioner finding time for reading. Obviously, they know from experience and feed-back from patients, the good and bad points from most drugs, but with so many side effects one wonders where it will end.

We come back to the common sense explanation that dis-ease is the result of something wrong deep in the economy of the person, probably triggered off by one of the mind-states. Physical troubles are the outward manifestation of this "hidden" illness. Mind symptoms are signs that there is something wrong within — and because each patient reacts differently we need to be treated with different remedies.

14

I have tried to give a few examples of the many mind states with which homoeopathy can deal, and without any side-effects whatsoever.

ANXIETY

Anxiety is the great modern plague
                        Smiley Branton, M.D.

What exactly do we mean by anxiety? Most people find this very difficult to explain although many know what it feels like to be anxious or worried, and I am dealing with anxiety and worry together because I think that the two are synonymous.

It is so strange that, generally, people are much more willing to relate their anxieties and worries than they are to tell about happy experiences, and so often then end up by saying "in fact I'm sick with worry". This can be true literally because a strong emotion like anxiety will, in time, cause physical conditions to appear and sometimes vomiting occurs.

There are endless causes of anxiety and worry. Anticipating an event – an examination, driving test or even getting ready for something enjoyable like giving a dinner party can cause great anxiety and a het-up state of mind.

Many people worry about illness and we all know the mother who has many anxieties about her grown up family, even if they are married and live away from home. Many patients have said to me "Of course I'm always thinking of my daughter and get very anxious if she does not let me know that she and her family are all right."

Many older people get into anxious states about the future. The list is endless and the minds of all these people go round and round creating many problems. I cannot remember who said "People borrow troubles" but what a true saying that is.

Some years ago I listened to an acquaintance who was in a very het-up state telling me a long story of woe. When I could get a word in I said "do try and stop worrying before you make yourself ill. Worry will never solve your problems but it **will** damage your health." She looked at me in absolute astonishment and said "But I was born a worrier and my mother worried about everything". That was the end of the conversation because I knew her sufficiently to realize that it would take a very long time to change her views or come round to homoeopathy.

Tranquillising drugs may dampen down the anxious and worried feelings but they do nothing to remove them.

On the other hand, from the great choice of homoeopathic remedies, one which matches the symptoms of the patient can usually be found and it will bring back feelings of joyous living once more and that is what life is all about.

FEAR

Fear, the opposite of boldness, is the most paralyzing of all emotions. It can literally stiffen the muscles and it can also stupify the mind and the will.   Arthur Gordon

Fear can be a very strong emotion that produces all kinds of symptoms; there are many fears, and some develop into terror.

If we are honest, I think we have to confess that we are all fearful of something yet we all react to fear in many different ways.

A friend of mine has a great fear of spiders. If she saw one in her bungalow she would panic, literally, and end up by feeling ill. That was after somebody (and she would ask anybody if she was alone) had removed it to the garden.

I was shocked not long ago when I had to move from the edge of the pavement in the main shopping street in Tavistock where two women were chatting. One had a pram which held a lovely fair-headed child of about two, she had fine features and pale pink cheeks. Just at that moment an enormous lorry rumbled past, the road is not very wide and it came near to the pram which was on the curb. The face of that little girl wrinkled up in fear and she seemed to shrink in size. A second vehicle followed – the noise was deafening – she cringed again, the two lorries must have seemed very large indeed to her. She didn't cry but I could "feel" her terror as I passed by. Her mother went on chatting and was quite oblivious of the child's fright. Obviously she was a very sensitive little thing; it looked as though she was almost too frightened to cry, and I couldn't help thinking that her health could suffer at some future date if she got into that kind of state very often.

Anything that is bottled up inside causes lots of problems.

People living alone are often full of fears which seem to multiply as thoughts go round and round in the mind without resolving anything.

Fears about the future, of illness, that something awful may happen; of being left alone; of the dark; of burglars; the list is endless and each fear is very real to the person concerned.

The unfortunate thing is that reasoning with the patient or trying to explain the fear is nearly always unacceptable.

Intellectually they know that the explanation is right but they can do nothing about removing the fear – or so they think – and the Benzodiazepine drugs do nothing to remove it either, they merely dampen down the reactions of the patient for periods of time, and at the same time, in many instances start the reaction of side-effects.

Another aspect of fear which can cause a great deal of suffering is the fear that remains in the system and can be "re-lived", sometimes years afterwards, when something triggers off a series of events or train of thought which brings it back into the mind. This re-lived fear is just as vivid and difficult to cope with as it was the first time round. I have had many patients who have come for the treatment of widely differing symptoms which I have been able to pin-point to a resurrected fear from the past.

There are many homoeopathic remedies which have helped patients to cope with problems of fear, including opium which is often prescribed for fears that remain and are re-lived.

Quiet minds cannot be perplexed or frightened, but go on in fortune or misfortune at their own private pace, like a clock in a thunderstorm.

Robert Louis Stevenson

GRIEF

Faith draws the poison from every grief, takes the sting from every loss and quenches the fire of every pain, and only faith can do it.

J. C. Holland

Grief comes to all of us at some time in our lives and, as always, we react to it in many different ways because we are all different.

18

The loss of a loved one must surely account for most grief; and it can, of course, be devastating.

The worst thing that anybody can do in this kind of situation is to stay motionless and lock it all up inside without shedding a tear.

The "stiff upper-lip" of the Victorians did nothing to contribute to good health. "I was not allowed to cry" we hear very elderly people say, and in the past, showing emotions in public was frowned upon, and even to-day among some people any showing of the emotions is unacceptable.

Some people don't weep even in private after grief and this means that probably all their pent up emotions will create symptoms later on; they may not develop until some time after the event, and the "cause of the effect" are often not connected.

Many people do have a good cry in times of grief which helps to rid the system of much emotion. Here again we can differ. Some people "break down" and weep anywhere, at any time; others wait until they are in the privacy of their own home or room before doing so.

It is not unknown for hysteria to take over — this is more likely after a sudden death or shock.

The wife who takes tranquillisers after the death of her husband rarely comes to terms with the situation. They are not the answer.

Homoeopathy has remedies for all these states but each patient must be treated according to his symptoms. Ignatia plays a very important part in helping patients to overcome and control their grief. I cannot tell you how many times people have said to me "I don't think I could have got through the funeral without that wonderful remedy." It was very often Ignatia.

Natrum Muriaticum is another that is very helpful in these circumstances but other remedies do what is necessary if the symptoms match those of the patient.

Never let yourself become discouraged. Never give in to a negative; as easy as that may be to do. Remind yourself of the power you have, the power of faith.   Frotz Kunkel

MENTAL DEPRESSION

Nothing is more highly prized than the value of each day.   Johann W. Von Goethe

"I feel so depressed" is heard quite often in a busy practice and sometimes the patient cannot say why he feels as he does or what has caused the depression.

There are many causes. I have met many people (both men and women) who became depressed in retirement because suddenly there are great gaps in the day when they could find nothing to do.

Deep depression can follow a viral infection although if it is treated homoeopathically the patient will have no bad "after effects."

Many women suffer from depression at the time of the menopause, and others when much younger can become depressed after childbirth.

I have known patients who threaten suicide because of depression. Threats of this kind are not to be taken lightly though, thankfully, very few people try to or do take their own lives. Fortunately we have "suicidal" remedies which are prescribed when necessary and these, I think, highlight more than most, the great courage of the provers who have taken a substance until they have felt like commiting suicide. It is thanks to them that we can help people to come out of this depth of despair.

Mental depression takes on many forms. The most common is probably the patient who is sullen, disinclined to talk and from whom it is most difficult to extract any helpful information. Any mental exertion seems to make him worse and concentration is difficult.

And the patient who will repeat himself over and over again is not much better. The mind seems to be so dull and there is no spark to give it life.

But these states, of course, are symptoms in themselves. We have remedies under the heading "Indisposed to talk" for instance, and others under "Morose" and "Moody"; we are well equiped to help patients with mental depression.

Anti-depressant drugs may palliate for a time but they do nothing to cure the depression.

Homoeopaths probe for the cause which has triggered off the sad path of mental depression. But even if we cannot bring this to light, the totality of the symptoms of the patient will point to the most similar remedy and so the road to cure will be in sight.

Most people are about as happy as they make up their minds to be.   Ralph Waldo Emerson

The following states of mind can trigger off or add to those I have written about more fully, they can be part of any human make-up but should they become marked, then problems arise.

"Aversion to company" we accept and understand if the house is always full of people coming and going and there is very little, if any, peace and quiet. But if a person lives alone and does not wish to mix with other people, then

21

this can be damaging. We all needs friends at times and most of us are grateful for them. I have known couples who have lived almost isolated – "We only need each other" – and suddenly, one partner dies. The other is devastated, bereft of friends, and hardly knows how to go about making any. After a while depression, or something similar, creeps in and at this point one of the drugs that we have been discussing is often prescribed.

It is not abnormal to be indifferent to people we don't care about, or to things in which we are not interested. But, if this indifference is directed to loved ones, a member of the family or to a hobby, for instance, in which we have been very involved, then notice should be taken because something has gone wrong and the person concerned needs help.

Many people are restless and we sometimes say "I'm glad I don't have to spend too much time with her, she would be very tiring to live with" but it is said without rancour. We do though meet restlessness which is difficult to cope with when the mind of the patient is driving him and he cannot keep still. He sits down only to get up again to pace the floor or wander around; there is no peace of mind and no rest for the body. This is a terrible state for any family to have to deal with. Homoeopathy has a range of remedies to help this type of patient.

The last two states that I shall mention can really "eat into" the person concerned and cause terrible havoc.

The first is jealousy. Perhaps an immediate reaction is that we have all suffered jealousy, particularly when young and thought that somebody had pinched our boy/girl friend. That is very true but I am talking about the jealous person who is almost "green with envy."

I remember a woman I knew years ago who seemed to be jealous of everything; if relatives called wearing new clothes, or their children had new toys, terrible jealousy was written all over her face. She looked dreadful. She suffered many "bilious attacks" when she vomited green bile. I predicted that she would develop cancer at some later date. She died of cancer in her sixties. I feel sure that had she been treated homoeopathically for the "bilious attacks" when a full case history would have high-lighted all her weak spots, cancer would have been avoided.

And lastly suspicion. To be very suspicious is to have a mind that is very difficult to understand because the patient will not "come clean" when answering questions; he is mistrustful all the time. He is furtive and will go to great lengths to lead others "up the garden" and away from himself. In so doing, of course, he creates for himself more problems.

I hope these notes have given an insight into some of the conditions which homoeopathy can relieve and very often cure.

Chapter 4

THE MATERIA MEDICA

The following is a Materia Medica of 37 remedies which have been used in countless cases to clear up mind symptoms.

There are many more but in a book of this size the number had to be limited and these remedies have all done brilliant work in this field when their symptoms match those of the patient.

Each remedy is divided into 3 parts.

1. CHARACTERISTICS

There are several symptoms in most homoeopathic remedies that are extremely marked, e.g. the 4 to 8 p.m. aggravation of Lycopodium; the aggravation after sleep of Lachesis and the mid-morning aggravation of Sulphur – an "all-gone" sensation when he must have something to eat or drink.

We can "recognise" remedies from characteristic symptoms and so they help us to differentiate one remedy from another.

2. The second part of the remedy covers the mental or mind symptoms and this range over the 37 remedies covers a very wide field indeed.

These should be studied carefully.

Many remedies on the surface look similar and rather bewildering but the third section will prove very helpful in the choice of remedy.

3. MODALITY

This is a condition that modifies a symptom. It may be weather (better or worse from heat or cold); from motion (better or worse from movement or keeping still); the time of day or night when there can be an improvement or worsening of symptoms and so on.

Modalities are extremely important, they help us to get to know our remedies, and so choose the one that is indicated more easily.

To keep this book as simple as possible I have not included the physical symptoms of each remedy.

Small, full materia medicas are available but for our purpose I am sure all the relevant information is included in order that the remedy to match the patients symptoms may be found.

REMEDIES AND THEIR ABBREVIATIONS

ACONITUM NAPELLUS	*Acon.*
ANACARDIUM	*Anac.*
ARGENTUM NITRICUM	*Arg. n.*
ARSENICUM ALBUM	*Ars.*
AURUM METALLICUM	*Aur.*
BARYTA CARBONICA	*Bar. c.*
BELLADONNA	*Bell.*
BRYONIA	*Bry.*
CALCAREA CARBONICA	*Calc.*
CARBO ANIMALIS	*Carb. an.*
CAUSTICUM	*Caust.*
CHAMOMILLA	*Cham.*
CINCHONA OFFICINALIS (China)	*China*
COCCULUS INDICA	*Cocc.*
GELSEMIUM	*Gels.*
GRAPHITES	*Graph.*

HEPAR SULPHURIS	Hep.
IGNATIA	Ign.
KALI CARBONICUM	Kali c.
KALI PHOSPHORICUM	Kali p.
LACHESIS	Lach.
LYCOPODIUM	Lyc.
MERCURIUS SOLUBILIS	Merc.
NATRUM CARBONICUM	Nat. c.
NATRUM MURIATICUM	Nat. m.
NITRIC ACID	Nit. ac.
NUX VOMICA	Nux
OPIUM	Op.
PHOSPHORIC ACID	Phos. ac.
PULSATILLA	Puls.
RHUS TOXICODENDRON	Rhus. t.
SEPIA	Sep.
SILICA	Sil.
STAPHISAGRIA	Staph.
SULPHUR	Sul.
VERATRUM ALBUM	Ver.

ACONITUM NAPELLUS

Characteristics

Fear, anxiety, physical and mental restlessness.

Fright — Aconite has a calming effect.

The sudden beginning of an acute illness with fever, anxiety, restlessness and fear.

Fearful for the future, of death, there are so many fears.

Can vomit with fear.

There is much tension.

Compalints caused by exposure to dry cold winds and weather.

Tension is a keynote of Aconite; emotional and mental tension; inconsolable anxiety; great anxiety, often about illness and despair of being cured; palpitation with anxiety; internal anxiety; great agitation with anguish.

Very fearful; fears death; crossing the street;
misfortune; ghosts; the dark; to go out alone
after dark; fearful anticipation, particularly of
approaching death.

A strong disposition to be angry; to be frightened and to quarrel.

Moods changeable; can be sad, depressed,
irritable, full of despair; or excited, hopeful,
singing and dancing.

Restless; hurried; must move often.

Maliciousness.

Doesn't want to talk, mind feels paralysed,
weakness of memory.

Screams at slightest touch; slightest noise
intolerable; music intolerable; easily startled.

Very cross.

Predicts day of death.

Dreads some accident happening.

Anxious from fear, fright, shock and vexation.

Modalities
Worse: warm room; around midnight; cold,
dry winds, lying on affected side; music;
tobacco smoke.
Better: Open air.

ANACARDIUM

Characteristics
Loss of memory is stronger in Anacardium than
in any other remedy.

Pain in stomach when empty, better eating.

Pain and sensation as if a plug in different
parts.

Suspects everything and everyone around him.

Anxiety; apprehension; fearfulness; fears of
approaching death; fear and mistrust of the
future with discouragement and despair.
Despair of getting well.

When walking anxious as if being pursued.

Brain fag. Weakness of mind and memory, soon forgets things; absence of ideas; loss of memory.

Irritable; tendency to suicide; takes things the wrong way; contradicts; flies into a rage; screams; is furious and has to be restrained.

Hears voices; feels as if in a dream. Wants to swear and blaspheme when normally wouldn't do either. Feels he has two wills, each commanding or moving him to do opposite things — or one commanding him to do and the other not to do.

Has fixed ideas. Sees everybody's face in a mirror except his own; that a demon is sitting on his shoulder telling him offensive things; illusions, optical; of hearing; of smell.

Dreams vivid.

Modalities

Worse: On application of hot water.

Better: From eating; when lying on side; from rubbing.

ARGENTUM NITRICUM

Characteristics

Fear, anxiety, apprehension regarding future events.

Funks examinations.

Fears failure. Tummy turns over.

Irrational thoughts and imaginations.

Impulsive, does things in a hurry, walks fast.

Claustrophobia.

Looking from heights causes giddiness, looking up at high buildings also causes trouble. When in a theatre or other gathering seeks a seat which will enable him to make a quick exit or escape.

Dreads crowds.

Irresistible desire for sugar and sweet things which aggravate and cause diarrhoea.

One of the greatest remedies for anticipation; when preparing to go to church, or for an interview etc, gets diarrhoea; examination funk.

A leading symptom is great tremor, nervous feeling.

Nervous, especially at night with feeling of heat and fullness in head. Nervous, faint and tremulous feeling. Fears to be alone, thinks he is going to die.

Mental anxiety; very impulsive, must do things in a hurry but accomplishes nothing. Walks fast; hurries when going anywhere, fears he will be late.

Impulse to throw himself out of window.

Irrational, does strange things; fears passing a certain corner; fears high places, he might have an impulse to jump off; high houses make him feel dizzy.

Apathy; thoughts require effort; sluggishness in thinking.

Depressed, does not want to undertake anything in case he doesn't succeed.

Memory impaired, cannot find the right word.

Hysterical, nervous person.

Dreams horrid.

Modalities

Worse: Warmth in any form; at night; from cold food; sweets; after eating; at menstrual period; from emotion; left side.

Better: From eructation; fresh air; cold; pressure.

ARSENICUM ALBUM

Characteristics

Great anguish and restlessness.

Fear, fright and worry.

Prostration yet marked restlessness from anxiety making patient change places constantly.

Great exhaustion after slightest exertion.

Fastidious, hates disorder.

Burning pains better by heat but patient always want the head kept cool.

Burning discharges.

Great thirst for small quantities at frequent intervals.

Restlessness is one of the great characteristics of this remedy.

Anxiety; full of fear with restlessness compelling patient to frequently change position.

Anguish, driving her out of bed at night and from place to place in daytime.

There is irritability; great anger; despair; hopelessness; utterable misery.

Despair with anguish; despondency; weariness of life; inclination to suicide or excessive fear of death; despair of recovery.

Fearful of being alone; that things will injure him if alone; of going to bed; fear that something will happen.

Anger with anxiety, restlessness and sensation of coldness.

Ill-humour; impatience; vexation.

Apathy and indifference.

Repugnance to conversation.

Weakness of memory; stupidity and dullness.

Fastidious; exacting; fault-finding; violent.

Dreams of sorrow; fear; danger; fire; thunder; darkness; death.

Modalities

Worse: Cold air; wet weather; cold drinks or cold food; cold applications; night; after midnight; 1 a.m. to 3 a.m.

Better: Warmth (except head); loves and craves heat; from head elevated.

AURUM METALLICUM

Characteristics
Wants to commit suicide, thinks he is no good in the world.
Deep gloom and despair.
Over sensitiveness.
A great remedy for bone pains.

No remedy produces more mental depression than Aurum. A feeling of dejection; hopelessness; profound depression. Imagines that he is not fit for this world, longs to die. Sits apart in deepest sadness. Morose, indisposed to talk.
Discontented with himself, his circumstances.
Great anxiety.
Feels hateful and quarrelsome.
Aurum is also the greatest among the suicide remedies.
Mediates on death or suicide. Wants to destroy himself. Has no love for life, thinks he is worthless. Feels desperate. Thinks that all is against him and life is intolerable.
Despair of oneself and of others.
Complaints after grief, anger, disappointed love.
Hysteria, laughs and cries alternately.
Impulse to weep. Aversion to conversation.
Alternate peevishness and cheerfulness.
Grumbling; quarrelsome.
Weakness of intellectual faculties; weakness of memory.
Apprehension; full of fear.
Frightful dreams.
"Lack of gold has driven many to suicide; potentised gold has brought many back to life and hope."

31

Modalities
Worse: In cold weather when getting cold (many complaints come on only in winter), from sunset to sunrise.

BARYTA CARBONICA

Characteristics
Memory deficient; forgets in the middle of a speech. Great mental and bodily weakness.
Childishness in old people.
Sadness — dejection of spirits.
Timid; bashful; cowardly.
Dread of strangers.
Irresolute, constantly changing his mind.
Chilly people, need much clothing.
All symptoms are worse after eating.

Mentally and physically dwarfish; cannot grasp ordinary ideas.
Paralysis of mind and body; cannot be taught because cannot remember; great weakness of memory.
Lack of self confidence; aversion to strangers, or to society; shy.
Very anxious and fearful.
Irresolute; incessant activity.
Suspicious.

Modalities
Worse: While thinking of symptoms; from washing; lying on painful side.
Better: Walking in open air.

BELLADONNA

Characteristics
This remedy stands for HEAT, REDNESS, THROBBING and BURNING.
Attacks are violent and onset sudden.

32

Many acute local inflammations; fevers with hot, burning, dry skin, so hot that heat can be felt by the hand before it touches the skin.

Very red, flushed face; dilated pupils of the eyes.

Sudden rise in temperature.

Restless sleep from excited mental states which can go on to delirum.

There is often an acuteness of all senses.

Can get very angry.

Violence runs through all the "mental" symptoms of Belladonna. Depression and great agitation with continual tossing about; anguish (particularly at night and in afternoon). Desires to die; inclination for suicide. Excitement; delirium, raves, spits. Wants to bite, injure, strike. Twitches and screams out in sleep. Fears of imaginary things, wants to escape, run away. Anxious; nervous anxiety; easily frightened. Disposition to laugh, sing and whistle yet, at other times, great apathy and indifference. Desires solitude; dreads society; disinclination to talk.

Modalities
Worse: Touch; jar; noise; draught; after noon; lying down.
Better: Semi-erect.

BRYONIA

Characteristics
Complaints develop slowly.

Great irritability.

Excessive thirst for copious draughts at long intervals.

Stitching and tearing pains which are worse for any movement and better for rest.

Dryness of mucous membranes from lips to rectum.

33

Faintness when head is raised (sitting up in bed).
The Bryonia patient is worse from the slightest movement; and is worse from warmth.

Anxiety and restless with fear of the future; dreads the future
Anxiety about business; prattles about it.
Fearful with desire to run away.
Despair of being cured, with fear of death.
Aversion to conversation, wants to be left alone.
Very irritable and inclined to be angry. After anger he is chilly, has a red face and heat in head.
Memory bad.
Irascibility.
Great sense of insecurity.
In delusion thinks he is away from home and wants to go home.
"Do not cross a Bryonia patient, it makes him worse."

Modalities
Worse: Slightest movement; warmth; hot weather; cannot sit up, gets faint and sick; morning; eating; exertion; touch.
Better: Pressure; lying on painful side; rest; cold things.

CALCAREA CARBONICA

Characteristics
Fat; flabby; fair; faint.
A jaded state, mental or physical due to overwork.
Apprehensive and fearful.
Hand is soft, cool and boneless; gives you the shivers to shake hands with Calcarea.

Everything smells sour, stool, urine, and taste is sour.

Profuse cold, sour sweat, especially on head.

Sweats even in cold room.

Enlargement of glands.

Slow in movement.

Craves eggs and indigestible things like chalk, earth, raw potatoes.

Feels better when constipated.

Feet feel as if wearing cold damp stockings.

Great sensitivity to cold and cold, damp weather; dreads open air; at the same time cannot bear the sun.

Breathless; walking slowly up a slight hill can bring on sweating and breathlessness.

Fearful, has every kind of fear, that some misfortune may happen; fear about health, of death, of being alone, that she has some fatal disease; fear that she will lose her reason and that people will notice her confusion.

Great anxiety with palpitation.

Dread and anxiety for the future; dread and concern about imaginary things that might happen to her.

Anxiety and anguish; excited by fancies or frightful stories.

Shuddering and dread as evening approaches; sees visions on closing eyes. Aversion to darkness

Anxious agitation forbidding rest.

Exertion or excitement brings on exhaustion.

Ascending creates great weakness (walking up the slightest incline).

There is agitation; easily frightened or offended; impatience; great excitability; ill-humour.

Repugnance to conversation; aversion to other people.

Disgust and aversion to all work.

Great weakness of memory; thinking becomes difficult.

Dreams horrible; fear of fantastic dreams during sleep.

Modalities

Worse: On waking; morning; after midnight; bathing; working in water; full moon; new moon; mental and physical exertion; stooping; pressure of clothes; open air; cold air; cold, wet weather; letting limbs hang down.

Better: After breakfast; drawing up limbs; loosening garments; in the dark; lying on back; from rubbing; dry, warm weather.

CARBO ANIMALIS

Characteristics

Great weakness, no energy.

The flow at period time always weakens so she can hardly speak.

Weak ankles (especially in children).

Easily sprained from lifting.

A remedy which has helped many old people who are greatly debilitated, but of course it can help others if the symptoms match.

Nostalgia. Mournful; feeling of isolation; tearful; avoids conversation.

Fear and apprehension, especially in the evenings.

Feeling of discouragement and despair.

Easily frightened; fearful in the dark.

Alternate feeling of gaity and gloom; or of irascibility and ill-humoured taciturnity.

Confusion of ideas and dullness, worse mornings.

Modalities

Worse: After shaving; loss of fluids.

CAUSTICUM

Characteristics
Intensely sympathetic.

Depression; apprehension; timidity; irritability.

Aches and pains with soreness, rawness and burning.

Paralysis of single parts, e.g. face, throat, vocal chords, limbs, from exposure to cold, dry winds.

Skin dirty white, sallow.

Fearful, especially at night. Full of fearful fancies.

Anxious; apprehension of impending misfortune.

Restless apprehension.

Nervous; timid.

Great anguish.

Taciturn and distrustful.

Quarrelsome.

Indisposition to work.

Absence of mind; tendency to make mistakes when speaking.

Modalities
Worse: Dry, cold winds; in fine clear weather; cold air; motion of vehicle.

Better: Damp, wet weather; warmth; heat of bed.

CHAMOMILLA

Characteristics
Frantic irritability — cannot bear it — whatever it may be!

Impatient; over-sensitive.

Whining restlessness; impatient; snappish.

Is bad tempered when she cannot get what she wants.

Inability to control temper.

Attacks of great anguish; agitation; tossing about.
Irritability very marked.
Is hyper-sensitive to every impression; to pain.
Driven to frenzy by pain; there is excessive sensibility of nerves, angry at pain.
Inability to control temper; cross; uncivil.
Wants something new every minute then discards it.
Mental excitement; cannot keep still.
Tendency to be frightened; quarrelsome; peevishness; ill-humour.
Absence of mind; averse to conversation.
State of stupidity and apathy to pleasure.
Complaints that come on after anger.

Modalities
Worse: Heat; anger; open air; wind at night.
Better: Warm, wet weather.

CINCHONA OFFICINALIS (China)

Characteristics
Debility and complaints after excessive loss of fluids; bleeding; periods; diarrhoea.
Haemorrhage can be profuse with fainting.
Periodical affections, especially every other day.

Broken down constitution from exhausting discharges (e.g. haemorrhage; periods too prolonged or too heavy; diarrhoea).
No desire to live; lacks courage for suicide.
Apathetic; dejected; indifferent; taciturn.
Extreme sensitiveness, cannot tolerate noise or excitement.
Extreme nervous irritation with slowness of ideas.

Contempt for everything.
Great anxiety and fear.
Disposition to hurt the feelings of others.
Prefers to be alone.
Discontent.

Modalities
Worse: Slightest touch; least draught of air; every other day; loss of vital fluids; after eating.
Better: Hard pressure on painful part; bending double; open air; warmth.

COCCULUS INDICA

Characteristics
Extreme irritability of nervous system.
Cannot bear contradiction.
Profound sadness.
Effects of night-watching.
Sensation of hollowness; emptiness.
Time passes too quickly. Slowness in thinking, worse after an emotional disturbance.
Sensitive to hot or cold air.

Great fear.
Anxiety sudden, as if he had commited a crime.
Anxious apprehension.
Easily frightened.
Takes everything the wrong way.
Preoccupation of mind; sits engulfed in thought.
Loss of will and power to make decisions.
Sad; grief; despair.

Modalities
Worse: Eating; after loss of sleep (night watching); open air; smoking; riding; swimming; touch; noise; jar; afternoon; menstrual period; after any emotional disturbance.
Better: When lying quiet.

GELSEMIUM

Characteristics
Affects more the nerves of motion, causing muscular prostration and varying degrees of motor paralysis.

Dizziness, drowsiness, dullness, trembling.

Tiredness, limbs feel tired; eyelids feel heavy.

Fearful; terrors of anticipation.

Apathy regarding illness.

Bad effects of great fright and fear.

Fear of appearing in public — anticipation causes diarrhoea. Fear of falling.

Mind sluggish; mental prostration; examination funk.

Cannot think or fix attention; cannot follow an idea for any length of time.

Dullness of mental faculties.

Tremor; wants to be held.

Lack of courage.

Wants to be quiet, to be left alone.

Great irritability, doesn't want to be spoken to.

Modalities
Worse: Damp weather; before a thunderstorm; emotion; excitement; bad news; 10 a.m.

Better: Bending forward; open air; continued motion; headache better by profuse urination.

GRAPHITES

Characteristics
Fat, chilly, costive.

Tendency to obesity.

Eruptions oozing thick honey-like liquid.

Nails thick and mis-shapen.

Intolerance of light, especially sunlight.

Always cold but craves fresh air; must be well wrapped up.

Anxious, changeable, wavering mood.

Dejection, sadness, profound depression, foreboding.

Miserably unhappy, much weeping; also weeping without cause.

Agitation, anguish and fear that some calamity would happen.

Anxious agitation with inclination to grief.

Anxiety about the future.

Agitation in the morning.

Timid, irresolute, with cautiousness and hesitation; unable to make up his mind about anything.

Absence of mind.

Susceptible to impressions.

Dread of work.

Modalities

Worse: Warmth; at night; during and after menstruation.

Better: In the dark; from wrapping up.

HEPAR SULPHURIS

Characteristics

Hyper-sensitive to all impressions; to touch, pain, cold air.

Tendency to suppuration.

Coughs when any part of the body becomes uncovered.

Feeling as if wind was blowing on some part.

Sweats easily on slight exertion.

Hypersensitivity runs through mind symptoms as well as physical; the slightest cause irritates.

Hasty speech.

An ache or a disagreeable sensation to an ordinary person would be intense suffering to the Hepar patient.

Anguish in the evening and night with thoughts of suicide.

Dejected and sad.

Very irritable; becomes wild and impulsive when disturbed.

Sudden impulse to stab, set herself on fire, do violent things; mania to set fire to things.

Imagines frightful things.

Great anxiety in the evening.

Starts from sleep as if about to suffocate.

Dreams of danger, anxiety, of fleeing from danger.

Modalities

Worse: From dry, cold winds; cool air; slightest draught; from touch; lying on painful side.

Better: In damp weather; from wrapping up head; warmth; after eating.

IGNATIA

Characteristics

A remedy of contradictions.

Mental stresses and strains from shock, bereavement, fright, etc.

Much grief; long sighs; sobbing; unhappiness.

Twitching, spasms or convulsions from depression, fright, emotion etc.

Great aversion to tobacco smoke.

Weak, empty sensation in stomach not relieved by eating.

Changeable moods. Nash says "Ignatia may justly be termed pre-eminently the remedy of MOODS."

The sighing remedy; of silent grief; sobbing; utterly absorbed in grief.

Unable to control emotions and excitement.

The emotional element is uppermost; hysteria.

Effects of long continued grief, bad news, unhappy love, misplaced affections, shocks, disappointments.

Nervous temperament; sensitive; easily excited.
Apprehensive. Rigid, trembling patients who suffer acutely in mind and body.
Great dread; fears she will have an ulcer in stomach; that thieves will break in.
The remedy of contradictions; the unexpected.
Moody; introspective; silently brooding; sighing and sobbing.
Depressed; tearful.
Does not like to talk, prefers to be alone.
Oversensitive to pain.

Modalities
Worse: Morning; open air; after meals; coffee; smoking; external warmth.
Better: While eating; change of position.

KALI CARBONICUM

Characteristics
Cannot bear to be touched.
Pains stitching, sharp, cutting.
Anxiety felt in the stomach.
Bag-like swelling in upper eyelids.
Sweat; backache and weakness.

Broken down, aged people who are anaemic.
Cannot bear to be touched; starts when touched very lightly.
Sweat, backache and weakness, has to sit down.
Anxiety easily frightened; shrieks about imaginary appearances.
Fears about her disease, that she cannot recover.
Despondent; alternating moods.
Irritable.
Never wants to be alone.
Never quiet or contented.

Obstinate.
Hypersensitive to pain, noise, touch.

Modalities
Worse: After coition; in cold weather; from coffee; about 3o'clock in the morning; lying on left and painful side.
Better: Warm weather, though moist; in the daytime; while moving about.

KALI PHOSPHORICUM

Characteristics
Prostration.
Want of nerve power.
Nervous dread.

This is a great nerve remedy.
Conditions arising from want of nerve power, neurasthenia, brain-fag.
Feels weak and tired. Prostration. Slight labour seems a heavy task.
Mental and physical depression. Indifference.
Morbid acitivity of memory; haunted by visions of the past.
Loss of memory.
Indisposition to meet people; extreme lassitude and depression.
Very nervous; easily startled.
Hysteria.
Night Terrors.
Perverted affection, cruel to husband, to baby.
Says she is eternally and irretrievably damned.
Weeps wringing her hands.
Weary of life and dread of death.
Shyness with excessive blushing.
Anxiety; nervous dread.
Lethargy.
Many symptoms brought on by excitement; overwork and worry.

Modalities

Worse: Excitement; worry; mental and physical exertion; eating; cold; early morning.
Better: Warmth; rest; nourishment.

LACHESIS

Characteristics

Insanely jealous and suspicious.

Loquacity.

Worse from sleep. Sleeps into an aggravation (no matter what the symptoms).

Worse left side, sometimes moving to the right.

Intolerance of anything tight, especially round neck or waist.

Concentration difficult. Delusions. Dullness of mind.

Grief; ailments from grief.

Hysteria.

Mental depression.

Worse exertion of mind.

Suspicious.

Depressed disposition.

Restless, uneasy, does not want to attend to business, would rather go out somewhere.

Mental work is best done at night.

Fearful of being poisoned; thinks he is being persecuted.

Ailments from fright.

Apathy; weakness of memory.

Timid.

Over excitement and excessive nervous irritability.

Religious insanity.

Derangenent of time-sense.

Great loquacity.

Jealous.

Sad in the morning.

No desire to mix with the world.

Nightly attacks of anxiety; sleepless from anxiety; short naps with frightful dreams.
Nightly delusion of fire.

Modalities
Worse: After sleep; left side; in the spring; pressure or constriction; hot drinks.
Better: Warm applications; the appearance of any discharge.

LYCOPODIUM

Characteristics
Intellectually keen but physically weak.
Upper part of body thin, lower part dropsical.
Very apprehensive — anticipation — before delivering address, lecture etc., but fine as soon as she gets going.
Likes to be alone but somebody in the next room or other part of the house.
Weeps when thanked.
Good appetite but a few mouthfuls fills up and she feels bloated.
Excessive accumulation of wind in lower abdomen.
Fullness; flatulence; distension.
Intolerance of tight clothing.
Symptoms begin on right side and often move to the left.
Red sand in urine.
Craves sweets.
Worse 4 to 8 p.m. (no other remedy has this as such an outstanding symptom).

Silent; depressed; peevish; despondent grieving mood.
Mind tired, forgetful; worried business men when times have been difficult, can't think.
Aversion to work, to undertake anything new.
Confused speech; confusion about everyday things.

Inability to remember what is read.

Loss of self confidence; dislikes company yet dreads solitude. Wants to be alone yet have somebody in the same house.

Distrustful; suspicious; finds fault with everything.

Arrogance, can be very haughty when sick.

Easily frightened, at everything, even a ring at the door.

Fears that something will happen; fears going to bed.

Complete indifference.

Dreams anxious, vivid, frightful, horrid.

Wakes up cross or terrified.

Modalities

Worse: Right side; 4 to 8 p.m.; from heat; warm room; hot bed; warm applications, except throat and stomach which are better for warm drinks.

Better: By motion; after midnight; from warm food and drink; being cool.

MERCURIUS SOLUBILIS

Characteristics

Mouth offensive; tongue large, flabby, shows imprint of teeth.

Salivation with intense thirst.

Profuse perspiration which does not relieve.

Trembling; weakness.

All symptoms worse at night.

Sensitive to heat and cold.

Hasty; hurried; restless; anxious; impulsive.

Sudden anger with impulse to do violence.

Feels some evil impending, worse at night, with sweat.

Feel as though he has committed a crime; as though he has no control over his senses.

Memory weak.

Mind won't work on cold, cloudy, damp days.
Slow in answering.
Loss of will-power.
Mistrustful.
Weary of life.
Fearful dreams; of falling from a height; of robbers; of shooting; of a flood.
Excessive sweating at night.

Modalities
Worse: At night; wet, damp weather; lying on right side; perspiring; warm room and warm bed.

NATRUM CARBONICUM

Characteristics
Great debility caused by summer heat.
Chronic effects of sunstroke.
Weakness of ankles.

Cannot think, difficult, slow comprehension.
Mental weakness and depression.
Forgets what he reads; cannot add up figures.
Confusion of mind.
Brainfag.
Great depression and apprehension.
Constant fear and foreboding.
Anxious and restless during thunderstorms.
Very sensitive to noise, change of weather and to the presence of certain individuals.
Worries.
Music aggravates.
Nervous and physical exhaustion.
Weakness of mind and body.

Modalities
Worse: Sitting; from music; summer heat; mental exertion; thunder storm; least draught; changes of weather; sun.
Better: By moving.

NATRUM MURIATICUM

Characteristics

Ill effects of grief, fright, anger.

Consolation aggravates; wants to be alone to cry.

Depressed; moody.

Very irritable.

Great weakness and weariness.

All mucous membranes dry.

Craves salt.

Very thirsty.

Psychic causes of disease.

Ill effects of grief, fright, anger, of unrequited affections.

Depressed, particularly in chronic disease.

Fearful that "something is going to happen."

Fears robbers, insanity, of dying, of losing his reason.

Anxiety as if he had done something wrong.

Is aggravated by consolation.

Wants to be alone to cry.

Tears with laughter.

Irritable, gets into a passion about trifles.

Awkward; hasty.

Dreams, anxious, vivid, frightening.

Modalities

Worse: Noise; music; warm room; consolation; mental exertion; sea-shore (can also be better at the sea); heat and cold.

Better: Open air; cold bathing; going without regular meals; lying on right side; pressure against back; tight clothing.

NITRIC ACID

Characteristics
Irritability.
Pains as from splinters.
Sticking pains.

Sensitive to noise, pain, touch, jar.
Anxious about illness.
Thinks of past troubles.
Mind is weak and wandering.
Irritable; hateful; vindictive; headstrong.
Fits of rage, despair, cursing.
Nervous; excitable; discontented with himself.
Fear of death.

Modalities
Worse: Evening and night; cold climate, and also hot weather.
Better: While riding in a car.

NUX VOMICA

Characteristics
Very irritable; fiery temperament; impatient.
Can get excited, angry, spiteful and malicious.
Very particular and careful people.
Easily offended; anxious; depressed.
Sullen; fault-finding.
Over-sensitive to noise, slightest noise; strong odours; bright light; music. Feels everything too strongly.
Quick in movement.
Very chilly and when unwell in spite of layers of clothing and hugging the fire, still feels cold.

Zealous, fiery temperament.
Very over-sensitive to noise, light, smell, contradiction, draughts; sensitive to all impressions.

Uncontrollably irritable; violent temper.
Takes things the wrong way; can be abusive.
Feels everything too strongly.
Great anxiety without particular cause.
Easily frightened; fears to be alone; fear of knives in case he should kill himself or others.
Suicidal but lacks courage.
Sullen; fault-finding.
Frightful or sad dreams. Wakes from troubled, busy dreams.

Modalities

Worse: Morning; mental exertion; after eating; touch; spices; stimulants; dry, cold weather.
Better: From a nap (if allowed to finish it); in evening; while at rest; in damp, wet weather; strong pressure.

OPIUM

Characteristics

All complaints are characterised by heavy sleep, most are painless.
Hot perspiration over whole body except in lower limbs.
Complaints from fear when the fear remains (e.g., relives the fearful experiences months or even years after the event).

Delusions.
Excitable.
Indifference.
Says she is not sick, has no symptoms even when very ill.
Most complaints are painless.
There is dullness of mind, insensibility, even coma. When aroused from this condition has a look of anxiety and fear.
Talkative.
Affected by sound, light, faintest odours.

Easily frightened; sees ghosts, frightful objects and is in great fear.

Thinks they are murderers, criminals and wants to run away.

Lightness of head in old people.

No mental grasp for anything.

Complaints from joy, anger, shame and sudden fright. And from fear when the fear remains.

Modalities
Worse: Heat; during and after sleep.
Better: Cold things; constant walking.

PHOSPHORIC ACID

Characteristics
Drowsy, apathetic, unconscious but can be aroused to full consciousness.

Grows too fast and too tall.

Great physical and mental weakness.

Listless; impaired memory; apathetic; indifferent.

Mind tired, cannot collect thoughts or find the right word.

Mental prostration.

Difficult comprehension; answers slowly or not at all.

Cause is often from effects of grief and mental shock.

Indifference; despair.

Delirium with great stupefaction.

Modalities
Worse: Exertion; from being talked to; loss of vital fluids; sexual excesses.

Everything impeding circulation causes aggravation of symptoms.

Better: From keeping warm.

PHOSPHORUS

Characteristics

Extremely sensitive.

Fearful of thunderstorms; being alone; of the dark; disease; death.

Very affectionate; they need it and give it, yet there can be an indifference.

Desire to be rubbed.

Much weakness and trembling.

Burning pains.

Haemorrhages bright and freely flowing.

Thirst for cold drinks which are vomited as soon as they become warm.

Nervous debility; great lowness of spirits; easily vexed.

Fearful, feels as if something is creeping out of every corner.

Fear of the dark; of being alone; of thunder; that something will happen; of death.

Fearfulness with great fatigue.

Fear and dread in the evening.

Anxious gloomy forebodings, about the future, during thunder storms.

Oversensitive to all external impressions.

Excitement produces all over heat.

Feels as if in several places, cannot get the bits together.

Loss of memory.

Brain feels tired.

Indifferent to loved ones.

Sympathetic.

Tendency to start.

May uncover and expose person.

Restless; fidgety.

Dreams vivid.

Modalities

Worse: Physical or mental exertion; twilight; warm food or drink; from getting wet in hot

weather; change of weather; evening; lying on painful side; during a thunderstorm.
Better: Heat (everywhere except in stomach and head); in the dark; lying on right side; cold food; open air; sleep.

PULSATILLA

Characteristics
The temperament is mild and gentle but anger can appear, and irritability.
Tears come very easily; inclined to silent grief.
Conscientious, hates to be hussled.
Loves sympathy and fuss.
Changeable in everything; in disposition (like an April shower and sunshine); pains wander from joint to joint; no two stools are alike, etc.
Pulsatilla feels the heat; they must have air, it makes them feel much better.
Cannot eat fat, rich food, it makes them feel sick.
Thirstless, even with a fever.

Mild, gentle, yielding disposition but can be very irritable.
Fearful; fear and rage in spells.
Sleeplessness causes great fear.
Afraid of everybody; fears evenings; to be alone; the dark; ghosts.
Sadness. Weeps easily; bursts into tears when spoken to, or when giving symptoms.
Great sensitiveness.
Likes sympathy; enjoys a hug.
Highly emotional.
No pleasure in anything; vexed about nothing.
Morbid dread of opposite sex.
Religious melancholy.
Easily discouraged; timid; irresolute.

Changeable, mentally and physically.
Mentally like an April day.
Contradictory.
Dreams confused, full of fright and disgust.

Modalities
Worse: Warm room; warm applications (cannot bear heat in any form); rich, fat food; after eating; towards evening; lying on left or painful side.
Better: Cool, open air; walking slowly in open air but pains of Pulsatilla are accompanied by chilliness; cold applications; cold food and drinks although not thirsty.

RHUS TOXICODENDRON

Characteristics
Extreme restlessness with continued change of position.
Great apprehension at night.
Cannot remain in bed.
Triangular red tip of tongue.

Extreme restlessness with continued change of position.
Anxiety; apprehension; fear of night.
Great apprehension at night, cannot remain in bed.
Listless; sad; thoughts of suicide; wants to die or drown himself but lacks courage.
Despondent.
Mental prostration.
Delirium with fear of being poisoned.

Modalities
Worse: During sleep; cold, wet, rainy weather; and after rain; at night, during rest; drenching; when lying on back or right side.

Better: Warm, dry weather; motion; walking; change of position; rubbing; warm applications; from stretching limbs.

SEPIA

Characteristics
Great indifference to family (to husband and often children) and friends.

Averse to work; loses interest in what she ordinarily loves.

Irritable.

Easily offended.

Anxious.

Dreads to be alone.

Nervous; jumpy; hysterical.

Weeps when telling symptoms.

Depressed.

Hates sympathy and weeps if it is offered.

Wants to get away to be quiet.

Weakness; weariness.

Pains travel upwards.

A 'ball' sensation in inner parts.

Faints when kneeling.

Feels the cold, must have air.

Gnawing hunger.

Craves vinegar and sour things.

Aversion to meat, fat and often bread and milk.

Indifference to those loved best; averse to occupation, to family.

Resigned despair.

Irritable; easily offended.

Discontented with everything. Does not care what happens; no desire to work.

Inattentive.

Causeless weeping; absence of all joy.

Filled with concern about health.

Very fearful and frightened of real or imagined evils.

Anxious towards evening.
Dreads to be alone; very sad; weeps when telling symptoms.
Miserly.
Indolent.
Anxious and frightful dreams.

Modalities
Worse: Late morning and evening; washing; damp; left side; after sweating; cold; cold air; east winds; sultry; moist weather.
Better: Exercise; pressure; warmth of bed; hot applications; drawing up limbs; cold bathing; after sleep.

SILICA

Characteristics
Want of grit — moral and physical.
Yielding; faint-hearted; anxious.
Very sensitive to all impressions.
Easily irritated over trifles; touchy and self-willed.
Fixed ideas.
Intolerance of alcohol.
Suppurative processes.
Under nourished from imperfect assimilation.
Feels the cold.

Want of grit, moral or physical.
Yielding; faint-hearted; anxious; nervous; excitable.
Mental weakness; brain-fag.
Nervous exhaustion.
Embarrassment; dread; hates disputes and arguments.
Dreads undertaking anything new.
Dreads to appear in public.
Dread of the future.

Dread that he will fail; wants to shirk everything; anything for a quiet life.
Sensitive to all impressions.

Modalities
Worse: New moon; morning; from washing; during menses; lying down; lying on left side; uncovering; damp; cold.
Better: Warmth; wrapping up head; in the summer; in wet or humid weather.

STAPHISAGRIA

Characteristics
Very sensitive.
Severe pain following abdominal operation.
Irritable bladder in young married women.
Scratching changes location of itching.
Backache, worse in morning before rising.

Ill effects of anger and insults.
Very sensitive to what others say about her.
Suffers from pride, envy, chagrin.
If suppressed anger and indignation is controlled she suffers.
If he has to control himself he goes to pieces.
Broods over old slight or injury.
Whole mind and nervous system in a fret.
Peevish; impetuous; violent outbursts of passion.
Hypochondriacal, sad; prefers solitude.
Dwells on sexual matters.
Ailments from indignation; vexation; suppressed anger.

Modalities
Worse: Anger; indignation; grief; mortification; loss of fluids; sexual excesses; tobacco; least touch on affected parts.
Better: After breakfast; warmth; rest at night.

SULPHUR

Characteristics

This remedy is known as the ragged philosopher.

Selfish, lazy and untidy people who often fling themselves into a chair with one leg draped over an arm.

Philosophical people wanting to know the "Why's and wherefore's".

Skin burning with itching, worse from warmth of bed.

Red orifices; eyes, nose, ears, lips and anus.

Sinking feeling mid-morning.

Worse standing.

Discharges offensive; acrid and excoriating, making part over which they flow red and burning.

Dislike of water; of washing.

Cat-nap sleep.

Anxiety; fear of misfortune; fear for others.

Untidy; full of theories; "the ragged philosopher".

Dwells on philosophical speculations.

Very forgetful; difficult thinking; answers irrelevantly.

Delusions, thinks rags beautiful; that he is wealthy; foolish happiness and pride.

Irritable.

Very selfish; no regard for others.

Averse to business; loafs around, too lazy to rouse himself.

Imagines giving wrong things to people causing their deaths.

Religious melancholy.

Depressed.

Thin and weak even with good appetite.

Vivid dreams of danger from fire.

Modalities

Worse: At rest; when standing; warmth of bed; washing; bathing; in morning around 11 a.m.; night; from alcoholic stimulants.

Better: Dry, warm weather; lying on right side; from drawing up affected limbs.

VERATRUM ALBUM

Characteristics

Cold sweat on forehead.

Collapse with extreme coldness.

Profuse, violent retching and vomiting.

On standing is tormented with frightful anxiety; the forehead becomes covered with cold sweat, he feels nauseated, even to vomiting.

Great anxiety.

Violence and destructiveness.

Mania with desire to cut and tear things, especially clothes.

Lewdness and lascivious talk, religious or amorous.

Is often silent but if irritated gets mad.

Religious frenzy; preaches; prays; despair of salvation.

Sullen indifference.

Aimless wandering from home.

Delusions of impending misfortune.

Cold sweat on forehead with anguish and fear of death.

Frightful dreams.

Modalities

Worse: At night; wet, cold weather.
Better: Warmth; walking.

Chapter 5

HOW TO FIND THE CORRECT REMEDY

First of all I will explain the use of the following lists.

"The Repertory of Characteristics" gives an alphabetical list of all the characteristic symptoms in the 37 remedies, and the remedy or remedies which have these symptoms.

e.g. under "Apprehension" *Arg.n.*; *Calc.*; *Caust.*; *Lyc.*; *Rhus t.*; all have apprehension strongly marked.

Under "Breathless ascending" *Calc.* is the only one.

I have explained under MATERIA MEDICA that the "Characteristic Symptoms" are very important and strongly marked. They are more important than remedies shown under "General Repertory" which follows.

Again, under this heading all the general symptoms of the 37 remedies are listed in alphabetical order with the remedy or remedies which have the symptom.

The "Repertory of Dreams" follows this pattern.

Then we come to the "Repertory of Modalities" which is in three parts: – General Symptoms; Weather Symptoms and Time Symptoms.

In each section there are two parts – Better (or ameliorated by) and Worse (or aggravated by).

e.g. under Better: –

Eating: *Anac.*; *Ign.*

means that the patient is better by eating and both *Anac.*, and *Ign.*, have this symptom.

This pattern is followed through the whole of the section "Repertory of Modalities".

The symptoms of the patient should then be written down under the following headings: –

1. LOCATION

This may be difficult as we are dealing with mind symptoms but write down any information if it applies.

2. SENSATION

Describe exactly how the patient feels in his or her own words, as fully as possible.

3. MODALITIES

These are very important because they describe what makes the patient feel better or worse, in other words they define the sensations. A modality might be better or worse for heat or cold; any time in the 24 hours; for movement; for food and so on.

The following two cases are examples to illustrate repertory work.

Case 1. A patient complained of not wanting to do anything, she couldn't be bothered; had a "couldn't care less" attitude. She felt worn out. The latest thing that developed was an indifference towards her family. She became very anxious and fearful and although she was indifferent to her family she couldn't bear to be alone.

MODALITIES: **Worse:** in the evening; after sweating; in cold air and in any dampness.

Better: by exercise; warmth of bed and after sleep.

The most important symptom should be chosen and in this case we will take "Indifference".

Indifference (from General Repertory)
Ars.; *Bell.*; *Chin.*; *Kali p.*; *Lyc.*; *Op.*; *Phos.*; *Phos.ac.*; *Sep.*; *Ver.*

Indifference (from Characteristic Repertory)
Phos.; *Sep.*

Anxiety (from Characteristic Repertory) *Sep.*

Fearful (from General Repertory) *Sep.*

MODALITIES: **Worse:** evening *Sep.*

Worse cold air *Sep.*

Worse after sweating *Sep.*

Better: exercise *Sep.*

Better warmth of bed *Sep.*

Better after sleep *Sep.*

The remedy needed in this case is *Sepia.*

Case 2. Patient complains of fear and anxiety; great apprehension before doing things; a very nervous person. She has many fears and hates heights, will not go near the edge of a cliff as she fears she will fall over. Always in a hurry; has a great longing for sweet things.

MODALITIES: **Worse:** at night; after eating a lot of sweet things; from warmth.

Better: in fresh air; cool weather.

For our Repertory work we will take Anxiety, Fearful, Apprehensive, Hurried.

Anxiety: *Acon.*; *Arg.n.*; *Ars.*; *Lyc.*; *Sep.*; *Sil.*

Fearful: *Acon.*; *Arg.n.*; *Ars.*

Apprehension: *Arg.n.*

Hurried: *Arg.n.*

MODALITIES: **Worse:** night *Arg.n.*

Worse warmth *Arg.n.*

Worse sweets *Arg.n.*

Better: fresh air *Arg.n.*

Better cool weather *Arg.n.*

The remedy needed in this case is *Argentum nitricum*.

You will note in the first case that there are 10 remedies listed under "Indifference" in the General Repertory but only 2 in the Repertory of Characteristics which is the most important.

Repertorising is eliminating all the time so now we work on 2 remedies *Phos.* and *Sep.* When we look at "Anxious" we find only *Sep.* and this remedy comes through all the other rubrics.

Case number 2 follows the same pattern.

The indicated remedy should be given in the 6th or 12th potency for 2/3 weeks when an assessment should be made. If there is some improvement it should be continued for another week, then stop the remedy as homoeopathic potencies continue to work for a long time; if after 3 to 4 weeks the patient still shows improvement allow the medicine to continue its work. If the patient shows signs of slipping back give 9 doses of the same remedy in the 30th potency; three doses per day for 3 days and then no medicine for another month.

If, however, very little if any improvement shows up after the first medication then the symptoms should be looked at again very carefully and re-repertorised. If a different remedy is found then the same procedure should be followed as outlined above.

A word of warning should come here. If after 2 remedies have been tried without success the patient should then be referred to an experienced homoeopath. Our remedies in potentised form are energies and it would be very unwise to take several over a longish period because all energy is indestructible and might blur the symptom picture, should an experienced homoeopath have to prescribe later.

It is very difficult to treat onself homoeopathically. We are too "close" to ourselves to see objectively before answering questions. But if an attempt is made then I do urge you to think before answering questions and be extremely honest.

I hope very sincerely that many people will derive great benefit from the homoeopathic approach for any of the mind symptoms discussed in these pages.

Chapter 6

REPERTORY OF CHARACTERISTICS

Affectionate: *Phos.*
Alone but likes somebody in next room: *Lyc.*
Anger: *Bell.*; *Nux.*; *Puls.*
Anguish: *Ars.*
Anticipation: *Gels.*
Anxiety: *Acon.*; *Arg.n.*; *Ars.*; *Lyc.*; *Sep.*; *Sil.*
Anxiety felt in stomach: *Kali c.*
Apathy: *Gels.*; *Phos.ac.*
Apprehension: *Arg.n.*; *Calc.*; *Caust.*; *Lyc.*;
   Rhus t.
Attacks violent: *Bell.*
Aversion to fat and meat: *Sep.*
Aversion to tobacco smoke: *Ign.*
Aversion work: *Sep.*
Bad tempered: *Cham.*
Backache worse morning, before getting up:
   Staph.
Ball sensation, inner parts: *Sep.*
Bashful: *Bar.c.*
Breathless ascending: *Calc.*
Cause – exposure to cold, dry winds: *Acon.*
Changeable in everything: *Puls.*
Childishness: *Bar.c.*
Chilly, cannot get warm even with more
   clothes and a fire: *Nux.*
Claustrophobia: *Arg.n.*

Cold always, but craves air: *Graph*.

Collapse with extreme coldness: *Ver*.

Complaints after loss of fluids: *China*.

Complaints develop slowly: *Bry*.

Complaints from fear, when the fear remains: *Op*.

Constipated, better when: *Calc*.

Contradictions, remedy of: *Ign*.

Convulsions, twitchings or spasms from depression, fright, emotions: *Ign*.

Cowardly: *Bar.c*.

Craves fresh air: *Puls*.

Craves indigestible things: *Calc*.

Craves salt: *Nat.m*.

Craves sour things: *Sep*.

Craves sweets: *Lyc*.

Craves vinegar: *Sep*.

Debility from loss of fluids: *China*.

Debility from great summer heat: *Nat.c*.

Depression: *Caust*.; *Nat.m*.; *Sep*.

Desire for sugar and sweets: *Arg.n*.

Desire to be rubbed: *Phos*.

Despair: *Aur*.

Discharges acrid: *Sul*.

Discharges burning: *Ars*.

Discharges excoriating: *Sul*.

Discharges offensive: *Sul*.

Distention, feeling of: *Lyc*.

Dizziness: *Gels*.

Dreads to be alone: *Sep*.

Dreads crowds: *Arg.n*.

Dreads the future: *Calc*.

Dreads imaginary things: *Calc*.

Dreads strangers: *Bar.c*.

Dryness of mucous membranes: *Bry*.; *Nat.m*.

Drowsy: *Gels*.; *Phos.ac*.

Dullness: *Gels*.

Eruptions sticky: *Graph*.

Excited: *Nux*.

Exhaustion: *Ars*.

Eyes, pupils dilated: *Bell.*
Face flushed: *Bell.*
Faint-hearted: *Sil.*
Faint sitting up in bed: *Bry.*
Faintness: *Calc.*
Faints when kneeling: *Sep.*
Fair: *Calc.*
Fastidious: *Ars.*
Fat: *Calc.*
Fault-finding: *Nux.*
Fear of being alone: *Phos.*
Fear of dark: *Phos.*
Fear of death: *Acon.*; *Phos.*
Fear of disease: *Phos.*
Fear of failure: *Arg.n.*
Fear of the future: *Acon.*
Fear of thunder: *Phos.*
Fear with vomiting: *Acon.*
Fearful: *Acon.*; *Arg.n.*; *Ars.*; *Calc.*; *Gels.*; *Phos.*
Feeling as if wind is blowing on some part:
    Hep.
Feet feel as if in damp stockings: *Calc.*
Fiery temper: *Nux.*
Flabby: *Calc.*
Flatulence: *Lyc.*
Food, few mouthfuls fill: *Lyc.*
Fright, ill-effects of: *Nat.m.*
Frightened: *Acon.*; *Ars.*
Fullness, feeling of: *Lyc.*
Funks examinations: *Arg.n.*
Gloom: *Aur.*
Grief: *Ign.*
Grief, silent: *Puls.*
Grows too fast and too tall: *Phos.ac.*
Grit, want of moral and physical: *Sil.*
Gnawing hunger: *Set.*
Haemorrhage profuse: *China.*
Haemorrhage, freely flowing: *Phos.*
Hand soft, cool, boneless: *Calc.*
Heights, giddiness: *Arg.n.*

Hollowness, sensation of: *Cocc.*
Hurried: *Arg.n.*
Hysterical: *Sep.*
Ill effects of grief, fright, anger: *Nat.m.*
Impatient: *Nux.*
Impulsive: *Arg.n.*
Inability to control temper: *Cham.*
Indifference: *Phos.*; *Sep.*
Intellectually keen but physically weak: *Lyc.*
Irresolute: *Bar.c.*
Irrational thoughts: *Arg.n.*
Irritable: *Bry.*; *Caust.*; *Cham.*; *Nat.m.*; *Nit.ac.*;
    Nux.; *Puls.*; *Sep.*
Irritable bladder: *Staph.*
Irritability of nervous system: *Cocc.*; *Sil.*
Jaded state, mentally and physically: *Calc.*
Jealous: *Lach.*
Lazy: *Sul.*
Loquacity: *Lach.*
Malicious: *Nux.*
Memory difficult: *Bar.c.*
Memory loss of: *Anac.*
Mental stresses and strains: *Ign.*
Moods changeable: *Ign.*; *Nat.m.*; *Puls.*
Motor paralysis: *Gels.*
Movement aggravates: *Bry.*
Movement slow: *Calc.*
Mouth offensive: *Merc.*
Mucous membranes, dryness of: *Bry.*; *Nat.m.*
Muscular prostration: *Gels.*
Nails thick, mis-shapen: *Graph.*
Nerve power, loss of: *Kali p.*
Nervous: *Sep.*
Nervous dread: *Kali p.*
Night watching, effects of: *Cocc.*
Nourished, under, from imperfect
    assimilation: *Sil.*
Obesity: *Graph.*
Offended easily: *Nux.*; *Sep.*
Orifices red: *Sul.*

Pains, burning: *Ars.*; *Bell.*; *Caust.*; *Phos.*
Pains cutting: *Kali c.*
Pains rawness: *Caust.*
Pains severe, following abdominal operation:
    Staph.
Pains and sensation of plug in different parts:
    Anac.
Pains sharp: *Kali c.*
Pains soreness: *Caust.*
Pains splinter-like: *Nit.ac.*
Pains sticking: *Nit.ac.*
Pains stitching: *Bell.*; *Kali c.*
Pains in stomach when empty, better eating:
    Anac.
Pains tearing: *Bry.*
Pains throbbing: *Bell.*
Pains travel upwards: *Sep.*
Pains wander: *Puls.*
Paralysis of single parts: *Caust.*
Particular, very: *Nux.*
Perspiration hot: *Op.*
Perspiration profuse, which does not relieve:
    Merc.
Philosophical: *Sul.*
Prostration: *Ars.*; *Kali p.*
Prostration muscular: *Gels.*
Pupils dilated: *Bell.*
Quick in movement: *Nux.*
Restless: *Acon.*; *Ars.*; *Bell.*; *Cham.*; *Rhus.t.*
Retching profuse and violent: *Ver.*
Sadness: *Bar.c.*; *Cocc.*
Salivation with intense thirst: *Merc.*
Sand red, in urine: *Lyc.*
Scratching changes location of itching: *Staph.*
Selfish: *Sul.*
Self-willed: *Sil.*
Sensitive: *Phos.*; *Staph.*
Sensitive to cold air: *Cocc.*
Sensitive to cold and damp weather: *Calc.*
Sensitive to cold and heat: *Merc.*

70

Sensitive to hot air: *Cocc.*
Sensitive to all impressions: *Sil.*
Sensitive to light: *Nux.*
Sensitive to music: *Nux.*
Sensitive to noise: *Nux.*
Sensitive to strong odours: *Nux.*
Sensitive to touch: *Kali c.*
Sensation of hollowness, emptiness: *Cocc.*
Sensitive, hyper to all impressions: *Hep.*
Sensitive, over: *Aur.*; *Cham.*; *Nux.*
Sinking feeling, mid-morning: *Sul.*
Skin burning: *Bell.*
Skin burning and itching: *Sul.*
Sleep, cat-nap: *Sul.*
Sleeps into aggravation: *Lach.*
Snappish: *Cham.*
Sourness of stool, sweat, urine, taste: *Calc.*
Spiteful: *Nux.*
Sprains easily from lifting: *Carb.an.*
Standing, worse for: *Sul.*
Sudden onset: *Acon.*; *Bell.*
Suicidal: *Aur.*
Sullen: *Nux.*
Sunstroke, chronic effects of: *Nat.c.*
Suppuration, tendency to: *Hep.*
Suppurative process: *Sil.*
Suspects everything and everybody: *Anac.*
Suspicious: *Lach.*
Sweat cold on forehead: *Ver.*
Sweat profuse, particularly around head:
    Calc.
Sweats, cold, sour: *Calc.*
Sweats easily on slightest exertion: *Hep.*
Swelling, bag-like in upper eyelids: *Kali c.*
Sympathetic: *Caust.*
Sympathy and fuss, loves: *Puls.*
Sympathy and fuss, hates: *Sep.*
Symptoms worse at night: *Merc.*
Tearful: *Puls.*
Temper uncontrollable: *Cham.*

Temperament mild: *Puls.*
Temperament gentle: *Puls.*
Temperature, sudden rise in: *Bell.*
Tension: *Acon.*
Thinking, slowness of: *Cocc.*
Thirst: *Ars.*; *Bell.*; *Bry.*; *Nat.m.*
Thirst for cold drinks, vomited as soon as
    warm: *Phos.*
Thirstless even with fever: *Puls.*
Throbbing: *Bell.*
Time passes too quickly: *Cocc.*
Timid: *Bar.c.*; *Caust.*
Tiredness, even eyelids heavy: *Gels.*
Tongue flabby and large: *Merc.*
Touched, cannot bear to be: *Kali c.*
Triangular red tip of tongue: *Rhus t.*
Trembling: *Merc.*; *Phos.*
Untidy: *Sul.*
Vomiting profuse and violent: *Ver.*
Washing, dislike of: *Sul.*
Water, dislike of: *Sul.*
Weak, empty sensation in stomach not better
    eating: *Ign.*
Weakness: *Merc.*; *Nat.m.*; *Phos.*; *Sep.*
Weakness of ankles: *Carb.an.*; *Nat.c.*
Weakness no energy: *Carb.an.*
Weakness mental and physical: *Bar.c.*; *Phos.*
Weakness from period: *Carb.an.*
Weakness with sweat and backache: *Kali c.*
Weariness: *Sep.*
Weeps when telling symptoms: *Sep.*
Weeps when thanked: *Lyc.*
Worry: *Ars.*
Yielding: *Sil.*

GENERAL REPERTORY

Abusive: *Nux.*
Agitation: *Acon.; Bell.; Calc.; Cham.; Graph.*
Alone, wants to be: *China; Ign.*
Alone, wants to cry: *Nat.m.*
Alone, never wants to be: *Kali c.*
Anger: *Acon.; Bry.; Cham.; Merc.*
Anguish: *Acon.; Ars.; Bell.; Calc.; Caust.;*
    Cham.; Graph.; Hep.
Anticipation: *Arg.n.*
Anticipation causes diarrhoea: *Gels.*
Anxiety: *Acon.; Anac.; Arg.n.; Ars.; Aur.;*
    Bar.c.; Bell.; Bry.; Calc.; Caust.; China.;
    Cocc.; Graph.; Hep.; Kali p.; Lach.; Merc.;
    Rhus t.; Sep.; Sil.; Sul.
Anxiety towards evening: *Sep.*
Anxiety about the future: *Graph.*
Anxiety great: *Nux.; Ver.*
Anxiety internal: *Acon.*
Anxiety with palpitation: *Acon.*
Anxiety felt in stomach: *Kali c.*
Anxiety during thunderstorm: *Nat.c.*
Apathy: *Arg.n.; Ars.; Bell.; Cham.; China;*
    Lach.; Phos.ac.
Apprehension: *Anac.; Aur.; Carb.an.; Caust.;*
    Cocc.; Ign.
Arrogance: *Lyc.*
Aversion to business: *Sul.*
Aversion to darkness: *Calc.*
Aversion to family: *Sep.*
Aversion to occupation: *Sep.*
Aversion to other people: *Calc.*
Aversion to society: *Bar.c.*
Aversion to strangers: *Bar.c.*
Aversion to work: *Calc.; Lyc.*
Awkward: *Nat.m.*
Brain-fag: *Anac.; Kali p.; Nat.c.; Sil.*
Brain feels tired: *Phos.*
Brooding silently: *Ign.*

Broods: *Staph.*

Cautious: *Graph.*

Changeable: *Puls.*

Cheerfulness alternates with peevishness:
   Aur.

Complaints following anger: *Aur.*; *Cham.*

Complaints following grief: *Aur.*

Complaints following disappointed love: *Aur.*

Complaints from anger: *Op.*

Complaints from fear, when the fear remains:
   Op.

Complaints from fright, sudden: *Op.*

Complaints from joy: *Op.*

Complaints from shame: *Op.*

Complaints painless, most: *Op.*

Comprehension difficult: *Phos.ac.*

Comprehension slow: *Nat.c.*

Concentration difficult: *Lach.*

Concern about health: *Sep.*

Confidence, loss of: *Bar.c.*

Confusion: *Lyc.*; *Nat.c.*

Consolation aggravates: *Nat.m.*

Constitutions broken down: *China.*

Contempt for everything: *China.*

Contradictions, remedy of: *Ign.*

Contradictory: *Anac.*; *Puls.*

Control, worse from: *Staph.*

Conversation, aversion to: *Aur.*; *Bry.*; *Cham.*

Conversation, avoids: *Carb.an.*

Conversation, repugnance of: *Ars.*; *Calc.*

Cursing, fits of: *Nit.ac.*

Darkness, aversion to: *Acon.*

Death, predicts day of: *Acon.*

Decisions, cannot make: *Cocc.*

Dejected, feeling of being: *Aur.*; *China*;
   Graph.; *Hep.*

Delirium: *Bell.*; *Phos.ac.*; *Rhusa t.*

Delusions: *Arg.n.*; *Bry.*; *Lach.*; *Op.*; *Sul.*; *Ver.*

Depression, mental: *Acon.*; *Arg.n.*; *Aur.*; *Bell.*;
   Graph.; *Ign.*; *Kali p.*; *Lach.*; *Lyc.*; *Nat.c.*;
   Nat.m.; *Sul.*

Derangement of time sense: *Lach.*

Despair: *Acon.*; *Anac.*; *Ars.*; *Aur.*; *Bry.*;
   Carb.an.; *Cocc.*; *Nit.ac.*; *Phos.ac.*; *Sep.*

Desperate, feels: *Aur.*

Despondent: *Ars.*; *Kali c.*; *Lyc.*; *Rhus t.*

Destructiveness of mind: *Ver.*

Discontented: *Aur.*; *China*; *Nit. ac.*; *Sep.*

Discouraged, easily: *Puls.*

Disposition depressed: *Lach.*

Disposition to hurt feelings of others: *China.*

Distrustful: *Caust.*; *Lyc.*

Dread: *Ign.*; *Sil.*

Dread of accidents: *Acon.*

Dread of appearing in public: *Sil.*

Dread of death: *Kali p.*

Dread in evening: *Phos.*

Dread of falling: *Sil.*

Dread of the future: *Bry.*; *Calc.*; *Sil.*

Dread of imaginary things that might happen:
   Calc.

Dread, nervous: *Kapi p.*

Dread of society: *Bell.*

Dread of solitude: *Lyc.*

Dread of undertaking anything new: *Sil.*

Dread of work: *Graph.*

Dullness of mind: *Ars.*; *Lach.*; *Op.*

Dwarfish, mentally and physically: *Bar.c.*

Embarrassment: *Sil.*

Emotional, highly: *Ign.*; *Puls.*

Emotions uncontrollable: *Ign.*

Examination funk: *Arg.n.*

Excited, easily: *Ign.*

Excitable: *Bell.*; *Nit. ac.*; *Op.*; *Sil.*

Excitement, uncontrollable: *Ign.*

Faint-hearted: *Sil.*

Fastidious: Ars.

Fault-finding: *Ars.*; *Nux.*

Feels things too strongly: *Nux*.

Fearful: *Acon.; Anac.; Arg.n.; Ars.; Bar.c.;
Bell.; Bry.; Calc.; Carb.an.; Caust.; China;
Cocc.; Gels.; Ign.; Kali c.; Lyc.; Nat.m.; Op.;
Phos.; Puls.; Rhus t.; Sep.; Sil.*

Fears to be alone: *Arg.n.; Ars.; Calc.; Nux.;
Phos.; Puls.*

Fear of appearing in public: *Gels.*

Fear of going to bed: *Ars.; Lyc.*

Fear of calamity: *Graph.*

Fear of crossing the street: *Acon.*

Fear of the dark: *Acon.; Carb.an.; Phos.; Puls.*

Fear of death: *Acon.; Anac.; Calc.; Nit.ac.;
Phos.*

Fear of disease: *Calc.; Kali c.*

Fear of dying: *Nat.m.*

Fear in evening: *Puls.*

Fear of evil: *Sep.*

Fear of falling: *Gels.*

Fear of future: *Anac.; Bry.*

Fear of ghosts: *Acon.; Puls.*

Fear of high places: *Arg.n.*

Fear of imaginary things: *Bell.*

Fear of insanity: *Nat.m.*

Fear of knives: *Nux v.*

Fears to be late: *Arg.n.*

Fear she will lose her reason: *Calc.; Nat.m.*

Fear of misfortune: *Calc.; Nat.m.*

Fear of night: *Thus t.*

Fear for others: *Sul.*

Fear of being poisoned: *Lach.*

Fear of robbers: *Ign.; Nat.m.*

Fear that something will happen: *Ars.;
Graph.; Lyc.; Nat.m.; Phos.*

Fear causes sleeplessness: *Puls.*

Fear of thunderstorms: *Phos.*

Fidgety: *Phos.*

Fiery temperament: *Nux.*

Foreboding: *Graph.; Nat.c.; Phos.*

Forgetful: *Sul.*

Frightened: *Acon.*; *Bell.*; *Carb.an.*; *Cham.*;
  Cocc.; *Kali c.*; *Lyc.*; *Nux.*; *Op.*
Furious: *Anac.*
Gentle temperament: *Puls.*
Grief: *Cocc.*; *Graph.*; *Ign.*; *Nat.m.*
Grief, ailments from: *Lach.*
Grief, effects of: *Ign.*
Grief silent: *Ign.*
Grit, want of moral: *Sil.*
Hasty: *Merc.*; *Nat.m.*
Hateful: *Nit.ac.*
Hates arguments: *Sil.*
Hates disputes: *Sil.*
Headstrong: *Nit.ac.*
Hopelessness: *Ars.*; *Aur.*
Hurried: *Acon.*; *Arg.n.*; *Metc.*
Hyper-sensitivity: *Hep.*
Hyper-sensitivity to pain: *Kali c.*
Hyper-sensitivity to noise: *Kali c.*
Hyper-sensitivity to touch: *Kali c.*
Hypochrondriacal: *Staph.*
Hysteria: *Arg.n.*; *Aur.*; *Ign.*; *Kali p.*; *Lach.*
Ideas, fixed: *Anac.*
Ideas, confusion of: *Carb.an.*
Ideas, slowness of: *China.*
Ill effects of anger: *Staph.*
Ill effects of insults: *Staph.*
Ill humour: *Ars.*; *Calc.*; *Cham.*
Illusions: *Anac.*
Imagines frightful things: *Hep.*
Impatient: *Ars.*; *Calc.*
Impetuous: *Staph.*
Impressions, susceptible to: *Graph.*
Impulsive: *Arg.n.*; *Hep.*; *Merc.*
Inattentive: *Sep.*
Indifference: *Ars.*; *Bell.*; *China*; *Kali p.*; *Lyc.*;
  Op.; *Phos.ac.*; *Phos.*; *Sep.*; *Ver.*
Indisposition to meet people: *Kali p.*
Indolent: *Sep.*
Insanity, religious: *Lach.*

Insecurity, feeling of: *Bry*.

Insensibility: *Op*.

Intellectual faculties, weakness of: *Aur*.

Introspective: *Ign*.

Irascibility: *Bry*.

Irrational: *Arg.n*.

Irrelevant answers: *Sul*.

Irresolute: *Bar.c*.; *Graph*.; *Puls*.

Irritable: *Acon*.; *Anac*.; *Ars*.; *Bry*.; *Cham*.;
    Gels.; *Hep*.; *Kali c*.; *Nat.m*.; *Nit.ac*.; *Sep*.; *Sil*.

Irritable uncontrollable: *Nux*.

Jealous: *Lach*.

Joy, absence of all: *Sep*.

Lascivious talk: *Ver*.

Lassitude: *Kali p*.

Lethargic: *Kali p*.

Lewdness: *Ver*.

Listless: *Phos.ac*.; *Rhus t*.

Loquacity: *Lach*.

Mad when irritated: *Ver*.

Mania: *Ver*.

Malicious: *Acon*.

Melancholy, religious: *Puls*.; *Sul*.

Memory bad: *Bry*.

Memory impaired: *Arg.n*.; *Phos.ac*.

Memory loss of: *Anac*.; *Kali p*.; *Merc*.; *Phos*.

Memory morbid activity of: *Kali p*.

Memory weakness of: *Acon*.; *Anac*.; *Ars*.;
    Aur.; *Bar.c*.; *Bry*.; *Calc*.; *Lach*.; *Merc*.

Mental excitement: *Cham*.

Mental faculties, dullness of: *Gels*.

Mental prostration: *Gels*.; *Phos.ac*.; *Rhus t*.

Mental weakness: *Nat.c*.; *Op*.; *Sil*.

Mild temperament: *Puls*.

Mind, absence of: *Caust*.; *Cham*.; *Graph*.

Mind, dullness of: *Carb.an*.; *Gels*.; *Op*.

Mind, worse exertion of: *Lach*.

Mind feels paralysed: *Acon*.

Mind, paralysis of: *Bar.c*.

Mind, pre-occupation of: *Cocc*.

Mind sluggish: *Gels.*
Mind tired: *Lyc.*; *Phos.ac.*
Mind wandering: *Nit.ac.*
Mind, weakness of: *Anac.*; *Ars.*; *Nat.c.*; *Nit.ac.*
Miserably unhappy: *Graph.*
Miserly: *Ars.*; *Sep.*
Mistrustful: *Merc.*
Moods alternating: *Kali c.*
Moods changeable: *Acon.*; *Graph.*; *Ign.*
Moody: *Lyc.*; *Puls.*
Morose: *Aur.*
Mournful: *Carb.an.*
Music intolerable: *Acon.*
Nervous: *Arg.n.*; *Bell.*; *Caust.*; *Ign.*; *Kali p.*;
     Nit.ac.; *Sil.*
Nervous debility: *Phos.*
Nervous exhaustion: *Nat.c.*, *Sil.*
Nervous irritability: *China*; *Lach.*
Nervous tremor: *Arg.n.*
Night terrors: *Kali p.*
Noise intolerable: *Acon.*
Nostalgia: *Carb.an.*
Obstinate: *Kali c.*
Offended easily: *Calc.*; *Sep.*
Passion, outbursts of: *Staph.*
Peevish: *Aur.*; *Cham.*; *Lyc.*; *Staph.*
Person may uncover and expose: *Phos.*
Prostration: *Kali p.*
Psychic causes of disease: *Nat.m.*
Quarrelsome: *Acon.*; *Aur.*; *Caust.*; *Cham.*
Rage: *Anac.*; *Nit.ac.*; *Puls.*
Religious frenzy: *Ver.*
Religious insanity: *Lach.*
Religious melancholy: *Puls.*; *Sul.*
Restless: *Acon.*; *Ars.*; *Bry.*; *Caust.*; *Lach.*;
     Merc.; *Phos.*
Restless in thunderstorm: *Nat.c.*
Restless very: *Rhus t.*
Sad: *Acon.*; *Cocc.*; *Graph.*; *Hep.*; *Puls.*; *Rhus t.*;
     Sep.; *Staph.*

Self-confidence, loss of: *Bar.c.*; *Lyc.*
Selfish: *Sul.*
Sensitive: *Cham.*; *China.*; *Ign.*; *Nat.c.*; *Nit.ac.*;
    Nux.; *Phos.*; *Puls.*; *Sil.*; *Staph.*
Sensitive to contradiction: *Nux.*
Sensitive to draughts: *Nux.*
Sensitive to impressions: *Nux.*; *Sil.*
Sensitive to jar: *Nit.ac.*
Sensitive to light: *Nux.*
Sensitive to noise: *China*; *Nat.c.*; *Nit.ac.*; *Nux.*
Sensitive to pain: *Nit.ac.*
Sensitive to smell: *Nux.*
Sensitive to what other people say: *Staph.*
Sensitive to weather, changes of: *Nat.c.*
Sensitive hyper, to every impression: *Cham.*
Sensitive over, to pain: *Ign.*
Sensitiveness, great: *Puls.*
Sexual matters, dwells on: *Staph.*
Shyness: *Bar.c.*; *Kali p.*
Sighing: *Ign.*
Slow in answering: *Merc.*
Sobbing: *Ign.*
Solitude, desires: *Bell.*; *Staph.*
Speaking, tendency to make mistakes when:
    Caust.
Speech confused: *Lyc.*
Speech hasty: *Hep.*
Startled easily: *Acon.*; *Phos.*
Stupidity: *Ars.*; *Cham.*
Suffers from chagrin: *Staph.*
Suffers from envy: *Staph.*
Suffers from pride: *Staph.*
Suicidal: *Aur.*; *Nux.*
Suicide, tendency to: *Anac.*; *Ars.*; *Bell.*; *Hep.*;
    Nux.; *Rhus t.*
Sullen: *Nux.*; *Ver.*
Suspicious: *Lach.*; *Lyc.*
Sympathetic: *Phos.*
Sympathy, likes: *Puls.*
Taciturn: *Carb.an.*; *Caust.*; *China.*

Talk, disinclined to: *Aur.*; *Bell.*
Talk, doesn't want to: *Acon.*; *Ign.*
Talkative: *Op.*
Tearful: *Ign.*
Tears with laughter: *Nat.m.*
Temper, inability to control: *Cham.*
Temper violent: *Nux.*
Temperament fiery: *Nux.*
Temperament nervous: *Ign.*
Tension: *Acon.*
Theories, full of: *Sul.*
Think, cannot: *Nat.c.*
Thinks of past troubles: *Nit.ac.*
Thinking difficult: *Calc.*; *Sul.*
Time, derangement of: *Lach.*
Timid: *Caust.*; *Graph.*; *Lach.*; *Puls.*
Tired: *Kali p.*
Touch, slightest, screams at: *Acon.*
Touched, cannot bear to be: *Kali c.*
Trembling: *Arg.n.*; *Ign.*
Tremor, wants to be held: *Gels.*
Untidy: *Sul.*
Vexation: *Ars.*
Vexed easily: *Phos.*
Vindictive: *Nit.ac.*
Violence: *Ars.*; *Bell.*; *Ver.*
Visions, sees on closing eyes: *Calc.*
Voices, hears: *Anac.*
Wandering aimlessly from home: *Ver.*
Want of grit, moral and physical: *Sil.*
Weakness: *Calc.*; *Kali p.*; *Nat.c.*; *Nit.ac.*
Weary of life: *Ars.*; *Kali p.*; *Merc.*
Weeping, much: *Aur.*; *Graph.*; *Kali p.*; *Nat.m.*;
    Puls.
Weeping without cause: *Graph.*; *Sep.*
Weeps easily: *Puls.*
Weeps when telling symptoms: *Sep.*
Work, indisposed to: *Caust.*
Worries: *Nat.c.*

Yielding temperament: *Puls.*; *Sil.*
Zealous temperament: *Nux.*

REPERTORY OF DREAMS

Anxious: *Acon.*; *Hep.*; *Lyc.*; *Nat.m.*; *Set.*
Confused: *Puls.*
Danger, fleeing from: *Hep.*
Danger, of: *Ars.*; *Hep.*
Darkness, of: *Ars.*
Death, of: *Ars.*
Disgust, full of: *Puls.*
Fear, full of: *Ars.*
Fear of fantastic dreams: *Calc.*; *Puls.*
Fire, of: *Ars.*; *Sul.*
Frightening: *Nat.m.*
Frightful: *Acon.*; *Aur.*; *Lach.*; *Lyc.*; *Merc.*;
    Nux.; *Sep.*; *Ver.*
Horrid: *Arg.n.*; *Calc.*; *Lyc.*
Sad: *Nux.*
Sorrowful: *Ars.*
Thunder: *Ars.*
Vivid: *Anac.*; *Lyc.*; *Nat.m.*; *Phos.*; *Sul.*
Wakens terrified by dreams: *Lyc.*

REPERTORY OF
MODALITIES

WORSE: –
Air, least draught of: *China.*
Alcoholic stimulants: *Sul.*
Anger: *Cham.*; *Staph.*
Bathing: *Calc.*; *Sul.*
Circulation impeded worsens symptoms:
    Phos.ac.
Clothes, pressure of: *Calc.*; *Lach.*
Coffee, after: *Kali c.*
Coition, after: *Kali c.*
Cold applications: *Ars.*

Cold drinks: *Ars.*
Cold food: *Arg.n.*; *Ars.*
Consolation: *Nat.m.*
Constriction: *Lach.*
Draughts: *Bell.*; *Hep.*; *Nat.c.*
Drinks, hot: *Lach.*
Eating: *Bry.*; *Cocc.*; *Kali p.*
Eating after: *Arg.n.*; *China*; *Nux.*; *Puls.*
Emotion: *Arg.n.*; *Cocc.*; *Gels.*
Exertion, mental: *Calc.*; *Nat.c.*; *Nat.m.*; *Nux.*;
    Phos.ac.; *Phos.*
Exertion, physical: *Bry.*; *Calc.*; *Kali p.*;
    Phos.ac.; *Phos.*
Excitement: *Gels.*; *Kali p.*
Fluids, loss of: *Carb.a.*; *China*; *Phos.ac.*; *Staph.*
Grief: *Staph.*
Jar: *Bell.*; *Cocc.*
Limbs, letting hang down: *Calc.*
Lying on back: *Rhus.*
Lying down: *Bell.*; *Sil.*
Lying on affected side: *Acon.*
Lying on left side: *Kali c.*; *Puls.*; *Sil.*
Lying on painful side: *Bar.c.*; *Hep.*; *Kali c.*;
    Phos.; *Puls.*
Lying on right side: *Merc.*; *Rhus.*
Meals, after: *Ign.*
Menstrual period: *Arg.n.*; *Graph.*; *Sil.*
Mortification: *Staph.*
Motion of vehicle: *Caust.*
Movement, slightest: *Bry.*
Music: *Acon.*; *Nat.m.*; *Nat.c.*
Noise: *Bell.*; *Cocc.*; *Nat.m.*
Perspiring: *Merc.*
Rest, at: *Rhus.*; *Sul.*
Sexual excesses: *Phos.ac.*; *Staph.*
Shaving, after: *Carb.a.*
Side, left: *Arg.n.*; *Lach.*
Side, right: *Lyc.*
Sitting: *Nat.c.*
Sitting up: *Bry.*

Sleep, after: *Op.*; *Lach.*
Sleep, during: *Op.*; *Rhus.*
Sleep, loss of: *Cocc.*
Smoke, tobacco: *Acon.*; *Staph.*
Smoking: *Cocc.*; *Ign.*
Spices: *Nux.*
Standing: *Sul.*
Stimulants: *Nux.*
Stooping: *Calc.*
Sweating, after: *Sep.*
Sweets: *Arg.n.*
Swimming: *Cocc.*
Talked to: *Phos.ac.*
Touch: *Bell.*; *Bry.*; *China*; Cocc.; *Hep.*; *Nux.*; *Staph.*
Uncovering: *Sil.*
Warm applications: *Lyc.*; *Puls.*
Warm drinks: *Phos.*
Warm food: *Phos.*
Warm room: *Acon.*; *Lyc.*; *Merc.*; *Nat.m.*; *Puls.*
Warmth: *Arg.n.*; *Bry.*; *Graph.*
Warmth of bed: *Lyc.*; *Merc.*; *Sul.*
Warmth, external: *Ign.*
Washing, from: *Bar.c.*; *Sep.*; *Sil.*; *Sul.*
Water, application of hot: *Acon.*
Water, from working in: *Calc.*
Wet, getting: *Phos.*
While thinking of symptoms: *Bar.c.*

REPERTORY OF MODALITIES

BETTER: –
Bed, heat of: *Caust.*
Bending double: *China.*
Bending forward: *Gels.*
Breakfast, after: *Calc.*
Cold applications: *Puls.*
Cold bathing: *Nat.m.*
Cold drink: *Puls.*

Cold food: *Phos.*; *Puls.*
Cold things: *Bry.*; *Nux.*
Cool, being: *Lyc.*
Dark, in the: *Calc.*; *Graph.*; *Phos.*
Discharges, appearance of: *Lach.*
Drawing up limbs: *Calc.*; *Sep.*; *Sul.*
Eating: *Anac.*; *Ign.*
Eating after: *Hep.*
Eructations: *Arg.n.*
Exercise: *Sep.*
Garments, loosening: *Calc.*
Head elevated: *Ars.*
Heat: *Phos.*
Hot applications: *Sep.*
Lying on back: *Calc.*
Lying on painful side: *Bry.*
Lying on side: *Anac.*
Lying on right side: *Nat.m.*; *Phos.*; *Sul.*
Lying quietly: *Cocc.*
Meals, regular, going without: *Nat.m.*
Motion, continued: *Gels.*; *Kali c.*; *Lyc.*; *Nat.c.*;
    Rhus.
Nap, if allowed to finish it: *Nux.*
Nourishment: *Kali p.*
Position,change of: *Ign.*; *Rhus.*
Pressure: *Arg.n.*; *Bry.*; *China*; *Nux.*; *Sep.*
Pressure against back: *Nat.m.*
Rest: *Bry.*; *Kali p.*; *Nux.*
Riding in car: *Nit.ac.*
Rubbing: *Anac.*; *Calc.*; *Rhus.*
Semi-erect: *Bell.*
Sleep: *Phos.*; *Sep.*
Stretching limbs: *Rhus.*
Tight clothing: *Nat.m.*
Walking: *Nux.*; *Rhus.*; *Ver.*
Warm applications: *Lach.*; *Rhus.*
Warm drink: *Lyc.*
Warm food: *Lyc.*
Warmth: *Ars.*; *Caust.*; *China*; *Hep.*; *Phos.ac.*;
    Sil.; *Staph.*; *Ver.*

Warmth of bed: *Sep*.
Wrapping up: *Graph*.
Wrapping up head: *Hep*.; *Sil*.

REPERTORY OF
MODALITIES

Weather

BETTER: –
Air, fresh: *Arg.n*.
Air, open: *Acon*.; *Bar.c*.; *China*; *Gels*.; *Nat.m*.;
  Phos.; *Puls*.
Cold: *Arg.n*.
Damp: *Hep*.
Damp wet: *Caust*.; *Nux*.
Humid: *Sil*.
Summer: *Sil*.
Wet: *Sil*.
Warmth: *Ars*.; *Kali p*.
Warm, dry: *Calc*.; *Rhus*.; *Sul*.
Warm, moist: *Kali c*.
Warm, wet: *Cham*.
WORSE: –
Change of: *Nat.c*.; *Phos*.
Cold: *Aur*.; *Kali c*.; *Kali p*.; *Nat.m*.; *Nit.ac*.;
  Sep.; *Sil*.
Cold air: *Ars*.; *Calc*.; *Caust*.; *Hep*.; *Sep*.
Cold dry winds: *Acon*.; *Caust*.
Cold wet: *Ars*.; *Calc*.; *Rhus*.; *Ver*.
Damp: *Gels*.; *Merc*.; *Sep*.; *Sil*.
Dry, cold: *Nux*.
Fine,clear: *Caust*.
Hot: *Bry*.; *Cham*.; *Lyc*.; *Nat.c*.; *Nat.m*.; *Nit.ac*.;
  Op.
Open air: *Calc*.; *Cham*.; *Cocc*.; *Ign*.
Spring: *Lach*.
Sultry, moist: *Sep*.
Thunderstorms: *Nat.c*.; *Phos*.
Thunderstorms, before: *Gels*.
Wet, rainy: *Rhus*.

Winds, dry,cold: *Hep*.
Winds at night: *Cham*.
Winds, east: *Sep*.

REPERTORY OF
MODALITIES

Time

WORSE: –
1 – 3 a.m. *Ars*.
3 a.m. *Kali c*.
10 a.m. *Gels*.
11 a.m. *Sul*.
4 – 8 p.m. *Lyc*.
Morning: *Bry*.; *Calc*.; *Ign*.; *Nux*.; *Sep*.; *Sil*.
Morning, early: *Kali p*.
Afternoon: *Bell*.; *Cocc*.
Evening: *Nit.ac*.; *Phos*.; *Puls*.; *Sep*.
Twilight: *Phos*.
Night: *Arg.n*.; *Ars*.; *Calc*.; *Graph*.; *Merc*.;
    Nit.ac.; *Rhus*.; *Sul*.; *Ver*.
Midnight, around: *Acon*.
On waking: *Calc*.
Moon, full: *Calc*.
Moon, new: *Calc*.; *Sil*.
BETTER: –
Breakfast, after: *Staph*.
Daytime: *Kali c*.
Evening: *Nux*.
Midnight, after: *Lyc*.
Night (when resting): *Staph*.

Chapter 7

OUR DAILY FOOD

Food is a great problem to many people suffering from conditions mentioned in this book.

Many patients have said to me "Oh, I can't be bothered about food" and on close questioning they have admitted that when tired or "fed up" they have a cup of tea and a cigarette. They rarely have a substantial meal but exist on snacks and easily prepared foods.

It should be understood that the nervous system is an integral part of the body and if health is to be maintained, it must be nourished by the intake of suitable foods.

I am not suggesting that anybody should become a crank or a food faddist, but common sense should be applied when catering, so let us examine some of the ways which will help overcome the "diet problem".

It should be borne in mind that each one of us is an individual and we all have our likes and dislikes, and there is no universal diet that can be recommended for everybody, because our needs vary.

The following advice is of a very general nature but the points stressed are important.

All "junk" foods should be avoided and a minimum of tinned and packaged items used;

when purchasing either, reject any containing additives, artificial flavours and colouring etc.

The consumption of meat should be limited. In some areas it is possible to obtain flesh of animals who have been reared on organic lines; that is to say they have fed on pastureland free of fertilizers and have not been injected with substances to induce un-natural growth.

More and more people realize the long term risks attached to foods grown in soil contaminated by artificial fertilizers. Meat from animals who have consumed food from that soil and who, also, have been injected with substances to increase milk yield to an artificial level cannot promote health.

Poultry and eggs should always be "free-range". Fortunately these are both more easily obtained than they were in the past.

Vegetarians have the advantage of no risks from animal flesh; I would therefore urge non-vegetarians to eat rather less meat and include some meatless meals in their diet.

There are many vegetarian cook-books on the market giving recipes for really appetising savouries which contain no animal products. I have given many friends, who normally enjoy meat, some of our favourite vegetarian dishes and they have been eager to take home the recipes because "we didn't know that vegetarian food could be so delicious".

A raw salad daily is beneficial for most people. Cooking, even conservatively, destroys many vitamins in food.

Salads can be exciting to make and pretty to look at. All kinds of things can be included in addition to the usual lettuce, tomato and cucumber. Almost any grated vegetable such as carrot, beetroot (raw, of course) and parsnip bring new flavours, plus onions, endive, watercress and mustard and cress. Nuts can be added, with raisins or sultanas, and any fresh fruit.

Whole-food cook books often include a chapter on salads, giving different combinations of flavours, which is helpful. Freshly picked herbs make a wonderful contribution to any salad.

Somebody once said "Milk is only good for baby cows"! We often hear of people being allergic to dairy products and I would suggest that milk be reduced to the minimum and semi-skimmed used. Otherwise, Soya milk is a good substitute. It can be obtained in several flavours for use with fruit etc., and I believe ice-cream can be made with it. The flavoured varieties contain brown sugar.

The less sugar we eat the better our health!

Sugar is very acid (especially refined white, castor or granulated) and it often causes digestive troubles. Large amounts of sugar can upset the nervous system as I have explained in Chapter 1.

Whenever possible honey should be substituted for sugar, but even this should be taken in moderation because, although it is a natural substance, it is still a sugar. Unrefined Barbados sugar is best, if it must be used.

Tea and coffee should be very limited. They are both real enemies if taken in excess; they can damage the nervous system and destroy natural vitamins and other elements in the body vital to health. Both drinks should be taken without sugar, honey can be used as a substitute but never resort to "sweetners".

Pure fruit drinks prepared from fresh fruit are excellent, they help to cleanse the system. There is a brand of bottled concentrated fruit juice available in Health Food Stores which is pure, as nothing is added; it is very concentrated so, although quite expensive, it goes a long way when diluted with water and it will keep for a reasonable time in the fridge, after being opened. There are several flavours, all with apple, and they are delicious.

Hot drinks for the winter are very good made from Marmite or Vecon. Also, they both make a very tasty spread on toast or in sandwiches.

Bread should always be made from 100% wholemeal flour as this contains the germ of the wheat and gives roughage. 100% self raising flour is also available; from this I make cakes, including sponges and biscuits. There is no white flour or sugar in my store cupboard!

For a long time there have been arguments about the merits of margarine versus butter. From what I have read and learned about margarine over the years I have always come up on the side of butter and providing butter is used in moderation (and in the context of whole food) I don't think it will prove very harmful.

Alcohol should be taken in strict moderation.

And lastly — aluminium pots and pans should never be used. Traces of aluminium can be found in all kinds of foods when tested in laboratories if cooked in aluminium pans and some people can be very allergic to it. Stainless steel saucepans are the best replacements; they are expensive but last for ever!! Oven-ware dishes too, are acceptable.

We are being warned about the dangers of cooking in micro-wave ovens. I sensed from the beginning that we should have adverse reports about them sooner or later. We don't really know what these waves will do in the long term apart from the fast cooking which is not natural. I suggest, therefore, that micro-wave cooking is suspended, at least until we are assured that it is completely safe.

Chapter 8

POSITIVE THOUGHT

Very little is needed to make a happy life. It is all within yourself, in your way of thinking.

Marcus Aurelius

I cannot finish this book without mentioning positive thought. The way we think is of the greatest importance, and has a direct bearing on our health.

All thought comes from the mind which uses the brain to control the chemistry of the physical body.

When we think positively, creatively, we are helping and healing ourselves. If we think negatively we harm ourselves because poisons are actually released into our bodies and every cell is affected.

There is a tremendous amount of negation in the thoughts of people suffering from problems of the mind. Negative thoughts seem to occur easily when we are ill.

Patients often worry a great deal about themselves, they cannot stop talking about their symptoms, and sometimes it seems as if the illness has taken over and they can think of little else. The thoughts are all negative; they can only worsen the condition.

But there is one thing that should never be forgotten.

WE ALL HAVE FREE WILL AND A CHOICE IN EVERYTHING.

I can understand the reaction of sick people when reading this; "but that is impossible, I'm ill and I cannot change".

But the point is we can all change; we all have the potential of health, and if we can say "I will try" we take the first step in the right direction.

I am not suggesting this is an easy exercise. Negative thinking has become a well-worn habit but if we really want to be different, slow and sure improvement will be made. The fact that the choice has been made, to try, will help.

Relaxation is all important.

This and the power of thought is discussed fully in three books mentioned in 'Books for further reading' and I warmly urge you to read them in order that you may help yourself with positive thinking.

USEFUL ADDRESSES

The Faculty of Homoeopathy,
(for the training of Doctors, Pharmacists, Dental and Veterinary Surgeons)
The Royal London Homoeopathic Hospital,
2 Powis Place,
Great Ormond Street,
London, WC1N 3HR

The British Homoeopathic Association,
27a Devonshire Street,
London, W1N 1RJ   01-935-2163

Homoeopathic Chemists

Ainsworth's Homoeopathic Pharmacy,
38 New Cavendish Street,
London, W1M 7LH   01-935-5330

Freeman's,
7 Eaglesham Road,
Clarkston,
Glasgow G76 7BU   041-644-1165

Galen Homoeopathics,
Lewell Mill,
West Stafford,
Dorchester,
Dorset DT2 8AN   Dorchester 63996

P. A. Janssen, M.P.S.,
The Pharmacy,
28 Ampthill Road,
Bedford MK42 9HG   0234 53484

Jolleys Pharmacy,
5 The Arcade, and 105 Witton Street,
Northwich,
Cheshire   0606 2663

Nelson Pharmacies Ltd,
73 Duke Street,
London, W1M 6BY   01-629-3118

Weleda Homoeopathic Pharmacy,
Heanor Road,
Ilkeston,
Derbyshire DE7 8DR   0602-309319

BOOKS FOR FURTHER READING

PERTINENT QUESTIONS AND ANSWERS
    ABOUT HOMOEOPATHY by Phyllis Speight
    (The C. W. Daniel Co. Ltd)

MEDICINE WITHOUT FEARS by Ken Derrick
    (The British Homoeopathic Association)

PUDDEPHATT'S PRIMERS by Noel Puddephatt
    (The C. W. Daniel Co. Ltd)

HOMOEOPATHY, A GUIDE TO NATURAL
    MEDICINE by Phyllis Speight (The C. W.
    Daniel Co. Ltd)

TREASURY OF COURAGE AND CONFIDENCE
    by Norman Vincent Peale (Unwin paperback)

WILL TO BE WELL by Neville Hodgkinson
    (Hutchinson)

LOVE IS LETTING GO OF FEAR by Gerald G.
    Jampolsky M.D. (Celestial Arts − California)